S0-CAJ-936

Waking the Tiger Within
How to be Safe from Crime

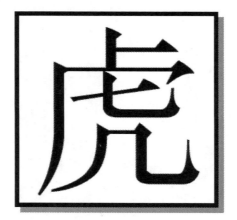

Waking the Tiger Within
How to be Safe from Crime

"Self-Defense that Saves Lives"

By
Scott Flint

Turtle Press   Santa Fe, NM

WAKING THE TIGER WITHIN: How to Be Safe From Crime. Copyright © 2001, 2008 Scott Flint. All rights reserved. Printed in the United States of America. No part of this book may be reproduced without written permission except in the case of brief quotations embodied in articles or reviews. For information, address Turtle Press, PO Box 34010, Santa Fe NM 87594-4010.

To contact the author or to order additional copies of this book:
Turtle Press
PO Box 34010
Santa Fe NM 87594-4010
1-800-77-TURTL
www.TurtlePress.com

Editor: Grant Flint
Illustrations: Chris Thompson
Photographs: Angelica Flint
Photo model: Katrina Flint
Author: Scott Flint

ISBN 978-1-934903-00-1
LCCN 2007049829
Printed in the United States of America
Fourth Edition

10 9 8 7 6 5 4 3 2 1 0

Library of Congress Cataloguing in Publication Data

Flint, Scott.
 Waking the tiger within : how to be safe from crime : self-defense that saves lives / by Scott Flint. -- 4th ed.
    p. cm.
 Includes bibliographical references and index.
 ISBN 978-1-934903-00-1 (alk. paper)
 1. Self-defense. I. Title.
 GV1111.F56 2008
 613.6'6--dc22
                        2007049829

WARNING

One of the main axioms of self-defense is to know what possible threats exist and find ways to prevent those threats from coming to fruition. I have spent most of my life gathering the information contained in this book, and I have devoted more than a year to committing that knowledge to paper. All this has been done for one reason, to help people. It is sad to think that in today's litigious society I might find myself defending against a legal attack from someone I was trying to help.

Because there are those who will misunderstand the teachings of this book, I must state the following:

This book is presented only as a means of preserving a unique aspect of the martial arts. Neither the publisher nor the author makes any representation, warranty or guarantee that the techniques and concepts described or illustrated in this book will be safe or effective in any and all self-defense situations or otherwise. You may be injured if you apply or train in the techniques of self-defense illustrated or described in this book, and neither the publisher nor the author is responsible for any such injury that may result. It is essential that you consult a physician regarding whether or not to attempt any technique described or illustrated in this book. Specific self-defense responses illustrated in this book may not be justified in any particular situation in view of all of the circumstances or under the applicable federal, state, or local law. Neither the publisher nor the author makes any representation or warranty regarding the legality or appropriateness of any technique or concept mentioned in this book.

Please e-mail questions and comments to: wakingthetiger@yahoo.com.

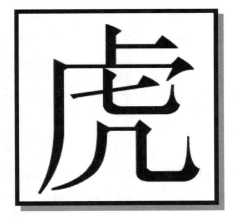

Quotes from Waking the Tiger Within

"This book will teach you simple steps designed to increase your awareness, develop your instinctual fighting ability, and give you basic common-sense techniques for keeping you safe while at home, at work, and while on the go."
PAGE ix

"Because you acknowledge the fact that you could be attacked, you are immediately more aware and that much less of a target."
PAGE xi

"If violence must be committed, let it be in your defense, and not to your demise."
PAGE xii

"No one ever has the right to hurt you. The mere thought of someone doing so should make your blood boil, and anyone who attempts to hurt you does so at his own peril.
PAGE 1

"You must be the Bazooka, not the B.B. Gun. So do everything in your power to avoid attack, but if it has to happen--strike hard, strike fast and end it on your terms."
PAGE 5

"Everyone is born with the tiger. Take heart in knowing that you have it, and with development from this book, it may someday save your life."

PAGE 19

"If the fight lasts more than three seconds, you are playing a game, and a deadly game at that."
PAGE 31

"If you have it firmly planted in your mind that, yes, if you are attacked, regardless of the odds you will fight back, then you will have acquired a new inner-strength, a new inner-peace, and you will have awakened the tiger within".
PAGE 136

TABLE OF CONTENTS

DEDICATION

This book is dedicated to the two people who have taught me the most in my life.

To my Dad, Grant A. Flint, accomplished author, teacher and father. You were the person who motivated me to start in the martial arts and who has continued to support me in every endeavor, including writing this book.

To my Sifu, Mr. Ron Lee, who taught me the Martial Arts, and through me perpetuates his system with this book.

ACKNOWLEDGMENTS

I would like to acknowledge all of the great students I have had the pleasure of teaching since 1978. Especially Mr. Chris Thompson and Mr. Jack Morris, both powerful leaders, excellent teachers, and the epitome of Black Belt.

Special thanks to Colonel Jeff Cooper who developed the awareness *Color Code* taught later in this book.

FOREWORD

My goal in writing this book is to pass on to as many people as possible the ability to live life without fear of attack.

Life is often short, and we should not let fear extort away our potential to lead happy, secure lives.

It isn't difficult to cultivate a way of life which keeps you safe and prepared for self-defense. This book will teach you simple steps designed to increase your awareness, develop your instinctual fighting ability, provide you with basic common-sense techniques for keeping you safe while at home, at work, and while on the go. You will also learn how to keep the children dear to you safe as they grow up, and what to do when terrorism strikes.

Throughout this text you will find reference to words such as goblin, dirt-bag, low-life, terrorist, burglar, kidnapper, abductor and attacker. To me these words all connote the same thing. (I do enjoy using the word *goblin* the most, because I feel it is the most descriptive). These terms all describe the sub-human, extra-legal vermin who take it upon themselves, for reasons that they feel sufficient at the time, to commit the heinous acts of: murder, rape, assault, home invasions, car-jackings, strong-arm robberies, kidnappings and an assortment of other evil deeds.

I feel that these creatures (I don't consider them human) are a blight on our society, and they will be the destroyers of civilization if left unchecked. Some will argue that these terms are designed to de-humanize these enemies of civility. **That's exactly why I have chosen to use them in this work.** I don't want you to think even for an instant that they are anything like you and me. For if you do, you will hesitate, or hold back in your defense against their attacks, thinking that their actions deserve "the benefit of the doubt." Once again, they are evil to their very core, and if you do hesitate, or hold back in your defense, **they will surely make you suffer for your compassion.**

Use your compassion to give more power and resolve in your defense. The compassion should be for your friends and family whose lives will be shattered should you allow the goblin to hurt or kill you.

The best way to use this book is to read what's being taught, always remembering the following concept: Imagine you found out without a shadow of a doubt that you would be brutally attacked sometime within the next thirty days. There was no way to escape from the attack. **It would certainly happen,** it was only a matter of when. What would you do? Your initial reaction would most certainly be fear. The fear of attack would cause you to prepare in every way possible. Once you felt prepared, **you would no longer need to be afraid.** You would then only need to be aware.

This book will make you aware of the possible threats that exist, which may cause you some fear. That fear will subside as each chapter teaches you new ways to be prepared. I hope that you will re-read each chapter five or six times before going to the next. By the end of this book, you need only be aware, for you will know what to do if attacked, and **you will be mentally set to take the action necessary to protect yourself.**

The aforementioned hypothetical concept of possible attack is not that far-fetched, for I can not guarantee to you that within the next thirty days, you won't be attacked. With 14,000 violent attacks happening every day in the United States, you stand a fairly high chance of one day becoming the target of a violent crime. What works against you is that every day you're not attacked, you start to think more and more that it won't happen, that you are somehow exempt.

It's easier to put your head in the sand and not think of being attacked, than to think of the possibility everyday and prepare for it. Violent crime is out of control because too many people don't want to think about it, don't prepare for it, and gamble that they won't be one of those 14,000 victims hurt or killed each day. I sincerely hope that **you will never gamble with your life in this manner.**

As our population grows, the chance of becoming a victim of violent crime increases. Not just because there are more attackers, but also because the pressure created by over-population causes more violent crime. **Unfortunately, it is only going to get worse before it gets better,** and our police forces, who are doing the best they can, can't be everywhere at all times. They are often only there to try to catch the goblin after the crime has been committed, which of course, is too late.

With an increasing population, your chance of having someone from a crowd help you when you are attacked, decreases instead of increases. Sociologists have studied this phenomenon and have come to the conclusion that it is caused by everyone in the crowd thinking the same thing: "There are so many people here, someone will step in and help, I'm not getting involved." There have been countless examples of large crowds watching terrible violent crimes, and no one in the crowd stepping in to help. If you are attacked, **you must only rely on yourself.** This book teaches you to be able to do that with confidence.

Some people will say that living by the principles this book teaches is too difficult, requiring too much time and energy; they say "I don't want to live like that."

They are under no obligation to do so. It's a choice. But, since you have made the **right choice** and are reading this book you have already reduced your chances of being attacked: because you acknowledge the fact that **you could be attacked,** you are immediately more aware and that much less of a target.

Most students who have learned and applied the principles of this book find that within a few weeks the concepts become second nature and are no more difficult than remembering to look both ways before crossing the street, or remembering to lock the door after coming home.

These concepts do take energy and thought to build into your life, but once you have them, you will be that much safer and happier for doing so.

In the past, I, as well as other martial art teachers, have been accused of promoting violence by teaching principles such as the ones contained in this book. The opposite is actually my goal, and more in line with reality. By using the following concepts and making them part of your life, you will become so aware that **no one will be able to get close enough to attack,** and because you will feel prepared to defend yourself, **you will repel instead of attract violence.**

If violence must be committed, let it be in your defense, and not to your demise.

This book has been purposefully kept as short as possible so that you can read it often. In the immortal words of a powerful warrior, Miyomoto Musashi, author of the Martial Arts Classic, *The Book of 5 Rings* -- **"Practice this often."** This was his famous adage to his students.

So I say to you, read this often, think of it always, and share this knowledge with the people you care about.

Be safe, be prepared,

Scott Flint

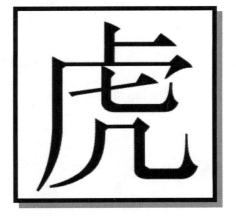

QUOTES FROM
THE RIGHT TO DEFEND

"The more prepared you are to fight, the less likely it will ever happen. **Be prepared.**"
PAGE 2

"If you are attacked by more than one assailant, it can be assumed that they have the collective ability and intent to cause you great bodily harm or death, and **you would be justified in taking them out.**"
PAGE 3

"Sometimes <u>thinking</u> <u>too</u> <u>long</u> about whether or not your action will be legally justified as self-defense--<u>will</u> <u>get</u> <u>you</u> <u>killed.</u>"
PAGE 4

"Keep in mind the law provides only for you to stop the fight. **You can not seek revenge or punish the goblin for his evil deed.** That is the province of the law and our judicial system."
PAGE 4

"**My advice is to trust your gut instinct. Don't hesitate.** First do anything to avoid the attack. If you are certain it's going to happen, take out the dirt-bag before he can ruin, or take away your life."
PAGE 4

CHAPTER ONE

THE RIGHT TO DEFEND

No one ever has the right to hurt you. The mere thought of someone doing so should make your blood boil, and **anyone who attempts to hurt you does so at his own peril.**

Your chances of being attacked are directly related to your level of willingness to fight back.

It's ironic that the more you prepare yourself to be ready to fight back, the less likely you will ever have to. This is an irony that is easy to live with, for you should never want to be in a position where you have to fight, and of course you should never "look for trouble".

Remember that no matter how proficient you become in the martial arts, there is always the chance of getting seriously hurt when you engage in violence. **It must always be the last resort.**

The best attitude to take in preparing for self-defense is to do anything and everything to avoid the fight, but if there is no recourse, you must *become your assailant's worst nightmare*--if you are to survive.

When teaching my students I like to call this way of thinking the **Bazooka** instead of the **B.B. Gun.** Meaning simply that if you engage in a fight you are prepared mentally and physically to **destroy** your assailant. The person with the B.B. Gun mentality thinks of fighting as a game, and approaches the conflict half-heartedly.

Try to imagine a person walking down the street with a B.B. Gun in his pocket being confronted by some low-life who bumps into him on purpose. The guy with the B.B. Gun would probably pull it out and shoot the low life, knowing that the B.B. would at most just hurt the guy. He would most likely use his weapon at the slightest provocation.

A person packing a Bazooka (a weapon designed to stop a tank), however, would understand that the use of his weapon would totally annihilate his attacker, and would only want to use it under a severe-threat situation.

I hope that after committing the principles of this book to heart you will become the **Bazooka,** and not the B.B. Gun. If you can view your self-defense abilities in this manner it will allow you to live a very non-threatened life, which will let you be more comfortable around others. And, because of the self-confidence it will give you, you will probably never be attacked. You will know in your heart that you are ready for the worst-case scenario where you have to defend your life.

Most beginning students are shocked when asking Black Belts if they have ever had to use their martial arts, because most often the answer to that question is: "The last time I got in a fight was when I was a beginner, because I was insecure and easily threatened."

Black Belts are constantly thinking of self-defense, and are totally aware of their surroundings. Attackers can feel this power and **will avoid this type of person like the plague.** Remember: The more prepared you are to fight, the less likely it will ever happen. **Be prepared.**

THE LAW

Laws vary widely from state to state and town to town, and it would take an entire book dedicated just to self-defense law to be able to give you all the particulars. It is in your best interest to check what the laws are pertaining to self-defense in your area. The following are **examples only.**

Your town or city may have very different laws and parameters governing self-defense. Once again, please take the time to check on them. It could make a big difference for you if you end up in court.

In many jurisdictions the law provides for you to take whatever steps are necessary to stop aggression directed at you, however, you are only allowed to use as much force against your attacker as he is using against you, and you must be able to prove to a jury of your peers that: 1.) **The goblin had the present ability to cause you great bodily harm or death,** and: 2.) **That he had the intent to do so.**   It can't be a future threat, like: "I'll kill you someday," or "I'm going to get you tomorrow." It must be a current threat that you can't get away from, and must act upon.

For example: If you are at a restaurant and you ask your waiter for a steak-knife, and as he approaches you with the steak-knife you hit him over the head with your chair, you won't be allowed the self-defense plea. The waiter may have had the present ability to cause you great bodily harm or death with the steak-knife, but he did not have the intent. If you were six-foot tall, and were approached by a four-foot-tall assailant who threatened to kill you, you wouldn't have the right to stomp him into the ground. He would not have the present ability to hurt you. On the other hand, if he pointed a gun at you, then you could take action, because he would of shown the intent to harm or kill you, coupled with the present ability (gun).

If you are attacked by more than one assailant, it can be assumed that they have the collective ability and intent to cause you great bodily harm or death, and **you would be justified in taking them out.**

Many times in court a woman who is being tried for hurting or killing a man who attacked her is more likely to be allowed the self-defense plea than a man in a similar situation. This is not sexism. Instead it is the result of the fact that often the male attacker is physically larger than the female victim. And it could be shown that he had the present ability to cause her great bodily harm or death. Her attorney would only need to prove that the male attacker had the intent to hurt her severely.

Sometimes **thinking too long** about whether or not your action will be legally justified as self-defense--**will get you killed.** I always think of the age-old adage: "I'd rather be tried by twelve than carried by six." What this means to me is: it's better to fight for your life and prove later why it was self-defense-- than to hesitate, get killed, and be carried by six pallbearers.

My advice is to trust your gut instinct. Don't hesitate. First do anything to avoid the attack. If you are certain it's going to happen, stop the goblin before he is able to hurt or kill you.

Keep in mind the law provides only for you to stop the fight. **You can not seek revenge or punish the goblin for his evil deed.** That is the province of the law and our judicial system. If while defending yourself you strike your opponent's eyes (blinding him), you have obviously stopped the fight. If you then chop his windpipe (killing him), you could be tried for man-slaughter or murder. It would be shown that you used excessive force.

The best mental set to use if attacked is *to be so focused on surviving that you literally don't care what happens to your attacker. All you want is to stop the fight.* If that means you yell **"Boo!",** and the creep runs away, then great! You stopped the fight.

You may end up at some time in your life fighting against an attacker you know. Not a stranger, but an acquaintance or even a close friend or family member. You are more likely to have to defend yourself against someone you know than you are against a complete stranger.

Defending yourself from the attack of someone you know can be very difficult. There is a strong tendency to hesitate, or to fight like the "B.B. Gun." The hesitation comes from thinking of the assailant as a friend, not as a foe. Many good people have been killed by attackers that they knew as family, friend or acquaintance. Ask any police officer what is the most common call that they get while on duty and they will respond, "Domestic disputes." (This is typically a fight between family members, often with deadly consequences). There have been thousands of reported cases of ex-boyfriends or ex-lovers coming back after a relationship has broken up to attack the woman that they theoretically once loved.

Get it in your head now that, yes, you can be attacked by someone you know. And if *anyone* ever tries to hurt you, regardless of who it is, you will fight back like a Bazooka!

You must be the Bazooka, not the B.B. Gun. So do everything in your power to avoid attack, but if it has to happen--**strike hard, strike fast and end it on your terms.**

Quotes from the Awareness Chapter

*"Make it a point to never let someone sneak up on you. Keep track of it.
See if you can go an entire month without anyone being able to surprise
you."*   **PAGE 8**

*"The bloodshed, the noise and terrible deaths overloaded their conscious
minds. Even if the victims had been armed, given their state of mind they
wouldn't have been able to return fire. They probably wouldn't even have
remembered that they had a gun."*   **PAGE 10**

*"Since you are reading this book, it can be assumed you have thought of
the possibility of being attacked. But get it in your conscious now, that it
really can happen to you. Unfortunately, no one is exempt."*   **PAGE 10**

*"No matter how well-trained you become in the martial arts, or the use
of a pistol, the club, pepper spray, etc., they are all useless if you can't
think to use them. Mental conditioning will take care of the catatonic
shock problem, allowing you to use your training effectively."*   **PAGE 11**

"Copy the tiger, walk with confidence, use your senses fully. Remember:
Awareness repels violence, fear attracts it."   **PAGE 12**

*"In orange, you make your battle plan. You say to yourself, "If he does
this, then I do that." You are setting the mental trigger that will put you
into action."*   **PAGE 14**

CHAPTER TWO

AWARENESS

The most important principle that you can get from this book is learning to improve your awareness level. It is the one major thing you can use to prevent being attacked, and you already have a built-in awareness system that is probably just not being used to its full potential. The purpose of this chapter is to strengthen this self-defense virtue.

Human beings are probably the most unaware creatures on earth when it comes to survival awareness. **This can be remedied.** You need look no further then your pet cat to see a perfect awareness model to copy. It is very difficult, if not impossible, to sneak up on your cat. This is because your cat is not consumed thinking of irrelevancies like: I wonder what's on T.V. tonight, or what kind of cat food do I like better, tuna or chicken flavor? Your cat is concerned, number one, with survival. **Do likewise.**

One good thing about the goblins that go around attacking people is that **they are inherently lazy, and don't want a challenge.** When they are scoping out their next victim, they are looking for someone that's easy. They are looking for the unaware. Unfortunately for society's sake, the unaware represent nearly 90% of people.

To prove this to yourself, pick a busy street, stand on the sidewalk and observe ten people walking by. What you'll probably notice is that only one of those ten will be observing you. The other nine will go plodding down the street, oblivious of your existence. Had you been a goblin, you would have been able to rob or attack any of those nine.

Which gazelle does the hungry lion go after on the Serengeti; The gazelle staring at the lion? No, the one with it's head down, grazing on the grass gets picked.

If you notice that people are continually catching you off guard, that you often run into people while rounding a corner, that you bump into things, that you have lots of near misses while driving then you're in very real danger of being attacked, because your awareness level is low.

Make it a point to never let someone sneak up on you. Keep track of it. See if you can go an entire month without anyone being able to surprise you.

Your size, your gender, where you travel, are all factors that determine how likely you are to be attacked. But they all pale in contrast to how important **your level of awareness is to your likelihood of being attacked.**

Science Magazine did a study in 1985, where they showed videos of different people walking down the street to a group of felons convicted of violent crimes. Four subjects were filmed. One was an older gentleman, the second was a man who walked with a severe limp, the third man walked with his head down in a depressed manner, the fourth man continually watched the person doing the video taping, and never took his eyes off the camera as he walked by.

Guess which subject was never picked as a potential target? That's right, the man watching the camera. When the felons were asked why they never chose him, they all responded with the same general comment, "He looked too confident, and too aware to take a chance on."

The other detriment to being caught unaware is not only are you going to be targeted for attack, but even worse, you can't respond to the attack in time, and will probably fall victim to your assailant.

The problem with trying to fight when you are caught unaware is the likelihood of slipping into catatonic shock. **Catatonic shock is a very common occurrence that has killed countless 1000's of violent-crime victims.**

Catatonic shock is the brain's reaction to being over-stimulated. The most dramatic example of this that I've seen, was from an old World War II news reel that showed the aftermath of the atomic bomb drops on Hiroshima and Nagasaki. The films showed hundreds of survivors walking down the burned-out streets, in a dreamy zombie-like state. The film crew and reporters would try to engage the Japanese people in conversation; they would snap their fingers in front of the survivor's eyes, or tap them on the shoulder, but received no response. They just kept walking slowly on as if the reporters weren't even there.

These survivors where in **catatonic shock.** They had only hours before witnessed things their brains just couldn't handle. First they saw an intense flash of light as the bomb exploded, then heard the terrible sound of the shock wave, louder than any sound that they had ever heard. Finally, the worst part came, the searing heat that vaporized friends and family members right before their very eyes. Their conscious minds could not handle it, and they shut down. Completely.

This same phenomenon happens all too often nowadays as people fall victim to violent crime-- for which they are in no way prepared.

A sickening example of catatonic shock in recent times was the famous "McMassacre" that happened in San Dimas, California. Scores of people were shot to death in a McDonalds. It was a classic case of everyone in the restaurant falling victim to catatonic shock.

A man trying to kill his wife (who he thought was in the McDonald's) fired shots into the restaurant before entering. Once inside, he proceeded to shoot and kill the diners as they sat frozen with fear, Big Mac's still in hand. Only two people got out. Two of the fast-food restaurant workers who saw the man outside the restaurant firing his gun had the presence of mind to run out the back door.

Only two of the diners inside the restaurant survived the assault. When interviewed, they both said the same sickening thing. *"I couldn't believe it was really happening. It was unreal, I was frozen, I couldn't think."* They survived only because a sniper finally took the gunman out. Given another few minutes, the gunman would have also killed those two.

Several times during the assault, the gunman ran out of rounds and had to change magazines--which took him around five seconds. In that time, **no one tried to rush the now defenseless gunman, nor did anyone attempt to escape.** They just sat there frozen, dumbfounded, as he took aim and continued his killing spree.

At another time during the goblin's attack, he turned away from his victims while he tuned in a song called "The Warrior" on the radio he had brought in. Once again, nothing from the "sheeple", who remained frozen in horror as he resumed his target practice.

Catatonic shock killed those people. Any person who was able to think clearly would have run out of that McDonald's the second they heard the gunfire. Definitely they would have fled while he was reloading, and without question when he turned his back to set the radio. That would have been the time to rush him, or to escape. No one did, and almost everyone paid the ultimate price for their non-action.

The violence in that restaurant was too severe for those people. The bloodshed, the noise and terrible deaths overloaded their conscious minds. Even if the victims had been armed, given their state of mind they wouldn't have been able to return fire. They probably wouldn't even have remembered that they had a gun.

Catatonic shock can be eliminated through two means. One is to heighten your instinctual level of awareness, and the the other is to learn **mental conditioning for combat.**

Mental conditioning works on the subconscious and has proved to work well under very stressful life-threatening conditions. The following system of mental conditioning was developed by Colonel Jeff Cooper from over 40 years of personal combat experience. **It is extremely effective and easy to learn.**

You simply say four phrases to yourself on a daily basis in order to condition your subconscious to be prepared for the unthinkable.

Number one: Every morning before you leave the house, you say, **"It might happen to me."** Meaning that you admit that you **really could be attacked. That you** *don't* **have an "exempt" sticker** on your forehead.

Since you are reading this book, it can be assumed you have thought of the possibility of being attacked. But get it in your conscious now, that *it really can happen to you. Unfortunately, no one is exempt.*

Second, you put the whole notion into a time context by saying: **"It might happen, today."** You are not just saying "Oh, I guess it could happen someday." You are saying, "Today could be the day I might have to fight for my life."

Third, you say, **"I know what to do."** After reading the chapter called the "Stop button" you will know what to do, and how to do it. As you say on a daily basis, **"I know what to do",** visualize fighting back, so your mind is used to the idea.

Fourth, and **most importantly**, you say, **"And I'm going to do it!"** You commit yourself before it happens, that if you are attacked, yes, **you will fight back.**

When these four phrases are repeated on a daily basis, they become a part of you, and you'll never hear yourself saying that sheepish: *"I couldn't believe it was really happening to me, it was unreal."* Instead you'll find yourself saying "Aha, I thought this might happen to me, **I know what to do, and I'm going to do it."** You'll be able to use the technique and tactics taught in this book to save your life, unhindered by catatonic shock.

No matter how well-trained you become in the martial arts, or the use of a pistol, the club, pepper spray, etc., they are all useless if you can't think to use them. Mental conditioning will take care of the catatonic shock problem, allowing you to use your training effectively.

Developing a heightened level of awareness is critical to avoiding an attack, and crucial to the defeat of your assailant.

Awareness must not be confused with paranoia or fear. When a tiger walks through the jungle on the prowl, he is not fearful or paranoid, he is aware. **He uses his senses fully.** His eyes scan from side to side, his ears move like radar to lock in on distant sounds, he smells the air around him, nothing escapes his detection. No creature dare attempt an attack, because the tiger is aware of them before they even get close.

Copy the tiger, walk with confidence, use your senses fully. Remember: *Awareness repels violence, fear attracts it.*

Colonel Jeff Cooper has developed over many years a time-tested means for enhancing your level of awareness. It is called **"The Color Code."**

The color code is comprised of four increasing levels of awareness marked by four different shades. They are: **White, Yellow, Orange,** and **Red.** Here is a break-down of what the colors connote, and how to use them:

THE COLOR CODE

CODE WHITE

UNAWARE, UNPREPARED, ASLEEP
WILL PROBABLY DIE IF ATTACKED

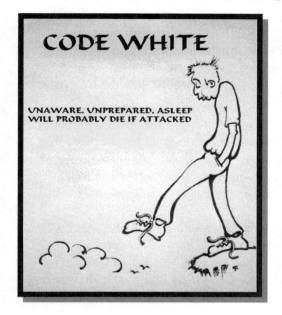

CODE YELLOW

AWARE, ALERT, CONFIDENT

DISCOURAGES ATTACKERS

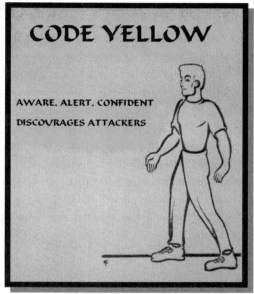

CODE ORANGE

FOCUSED ON A PROBLEM
MAKE DECISIONS
PREPARE TO REACT

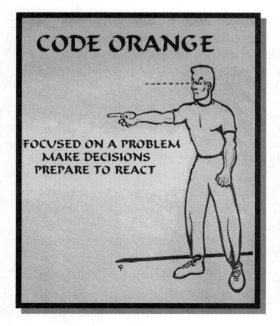

CODE RED
FIGHT MODE

DECISION ALREADY MADE

FOLLOW
THROUGH

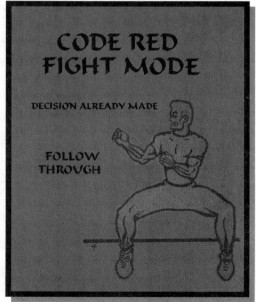

WHITE: Unaware, asleep, **you will probably die if attacked,** unless your opponent is a total moron who stabs you with the wrong end of the knife, or attempts to shoot you with an unloaded gun. In white, the only thing **that would get you to fight is the sight of your own blood.** Only then would you realize you've got a problem. 90% of people are in white most of their lives; it attracts trouble. **Don't ever let yourself be caught in white.** No matter how safe you think you are, **stay aware.**

YELLOW: General alert. You know you could be attacked, that **it really could happen to you,** that you are not exempt. You are aware of what is happening around you. You use your senses fully, you are living in the present and are focused on your personal safety.

Most of your life should be spent in this awareness level, especially when you travel to areas you are not familiar with. *You will repel attackers while in yellow* because as they look toward you as a possible victim you are looking at them as a possible attacker, and you are mentally and physically ready to deal with an attack. In yellow, you represent too much of a challenge.

Yellow takes effort to stay in, but **the effort is worth it** because it keeps violence away from you. If you are very tired, or feeling depressed, or you are sick with a cold or flu, you must make even a stronger effort to stay in yellow. **If you can't stay in yellow, consider not going out where you might put yourself in danger.**

ORANGE: Specific alert. You have a possible target. There is a particular situation that has drawn your attention, and could present a major problem. *In orange, you make your battle plan.* You say to yourself, "If he does this, then I do that." **You are setting the mental trigger that will put you into action.** You think to yourself: "If that goblin takes one more step toward me, I'll drive my fist into his throat." Or, "If he steps one step closer, I'll go into this store, and avoid the whole ordeal."

The importance of orange is that **you have made your decision to take action, and you have hung it on a hook.** Meaning "it is done." While being attacked **you won't have to have a conference with yourself on whether or not to fight back. That decision will have already been made,** and you will be able to fully concentrate on the matter at hand. **Stopping the fight.**

If while in orange, the potential attack situation does not materialize, you can then easily go back to yellow (the general-alert stage). This often happens, because when you shift into orange, and put 100% focus on your **potential attacker, he feels this readiness, and wants no part of you. Your willingness to take action defuses the situation.** If you were caught in code white you would most likely walk right into the attacker's grasp, resulting in a definite confrontation, and violence. *Orange puts you in complete control.* Your attacker will most likely feel this control and back down. If he doesn't, you automatically shift to color code Red.

RED: Red is the fight mode. It is where you carry out the decision you made in orange. Here, you are like a machine. **You don't have to think. The decision and course of action have already been made, and the execution of your technique will not be hindered by indecision.** You won't be saying, "I can't believe this is really happening".

You will not have been surprised. You will have seen the dirt-bag making his move toward you in yellow, established a course of action to follow in orange, and carried out that action in red. **The only person who will be surprised is your would-be assailant.**

Over the years we have had many favorable reports from our students on how well the color code works, and many have said it has **saved their lives.**

Just knowing and understanding the color code is not enough to make it an effective self-defense tool. **You must also practice it often.** This is actually quite simple to do. First, bypass white. **You should never find yourself in white.** Try shifting from yellow to orange often.

While walking down the street in yellow, practice imaginary shifts to orange. Say to yourself: "If that guy walking behind me picks up his pace, and makes a move toward me, I'm going to throw him through that store window." Most likely the guy walking behind you is not a problem, and when safe, you will shift back to yellow. Had he been a real problem, you would have been ready for action. Practice thinking of ways to stop, or avoid, potential attackers. Use anyone around you for mental practice.

Try to find yourself practicing this once a day. **Soon your ability to shift from yellow to orange will become effortless.** You can't really practice shifting to red, without it involving fighting. But you can imagine a shift to red by visualizing fighting-back in your mind. Once again, you are conditioning your mind to be ready to fight back. You are rehearsing for a performance that could determine whether you live, or die. **Make sure you know your part.**

Since Mr. Lee taught me the color code, I have tried to use it on a daily basis. I feel that it has kept me safe from countless potential threats. The following is one such example:

I recall in 1985 on a Saturday at around dusk, I was locking up the Berkeley Kung-Fu School after a day of teaching, and was headed for my car parked about one block away. As I walked to the car (my keys already in hand), I noticed some 50 yards away a guy across San Pablo Ave. at a diagonal to me, staring in my direction for no particular reason. I could barely make out his expression, but he looked to me to be angry, and focused on me.

Automatically I shifted from yellow to orange, and started to quickly formulate a course of action, as I said to myself, *"I thought this might happen, I know what to do, and I'm going to do it!"*

My plan was to continue toward my car while keeping a focused eye on the potential problem. If he made a move toward me I would speed up my pace, get to the car, and get out of there. If he got to me before I got to the car, I would launch an attack. I visualized striking his eyes first and then going for the throat.

So far, I was still in orange because he had not yet made a move, and only represented a possible threat. Then things changed quickly. Suddenly he was headed right for me at a good clip, moving on a diagonal across the very busy avenue, with no regard for the many cars that almost hit him.

I didn't know what he wanted, but my gut instinct sensed trouble I shifted to red, and carried out the plan. I sped up my pace to get out of there. He increased his pace to match mine.

I got to the car before him, got in, locked the door, started the car and put it in gear. As I was letting out the clutch, he grabbed on to the door handle, I punched the accelerator, leaving the dirt-bag in the dust.

To this day I don't know what he wanted, and I don't care. His facial expressions and body language spelled trouble. Because of the color code, I saw this all happening before it got out of hand. **The color code saved that dirt-bag.** Had I not been paying attention, I would have walked right into him, and under the circumstances, most likely would have killed him.

The color code saves lives. Try to practice it daily. Using it along with the mental conditioning spelled out earlier in this chapter, you will most likely not be picked as a victim. If you are you'll see it early, you'll make a plan of action, and you'll be prepared to carry out that plan if necessary.

Quotes from the Tiger Chapter

"You must attack all his senses, just as the tiger does. Communicate to him your severe hatred. Let him see it in your face, let him hear it in your shout, let him feel it from your strike." **PAGE 21**

"Most likely your assailant will not be thinking that you will fight back. He will be attacking you because he will have sensed fear, or weakness. *Surprise him with the tiger.* Your shout combined with the look of death on your face, should be enough to *communicate to him that he has made a grave error, and he'd better run for his life."* **PAGE 23**

"Powerful, passionate emotions trigger the tiger instinct." **PAGE 23**

"Fear and anger are very closely related emotions. Fear is a natural first-step emotion. What you must learn to do quickly, is to convert fear into anger. *The key is indignation."* **PAGE 25**

"A predator expects its prey to be fearful. *The fear triggers an instinctual green light for the predator to continue the assault.* If no fear is present, the predator will back down." **PAGE 26**

"It's O.K., and normal to have your first response to attack be fear, but you must instantly be able to turn the fear into anger and aggression. *Your assailant does not expect to deal with a tiger."* **PAGE 27**

CHAPTER THREE

THE TIGER

The name "Waking the Tiger within" was chosen to represent this self-defense book because it refers to the key ingredient needed in self-defense. This crucial ingredient is the fighting instinct that lives inside each and every one of us, without exception. **It is like a voracious tiger waiting to be let out of its cage.** *Everyone is born with the tiger.* It has been part of our nature since the beginning of man. Without it our species would have gone extinct, eons ago.

Though I have taught self-defense since 1978 and have worked with thousands of students, I have never come across a student who didn't have the tiger spirit. Some come into the school with the strength of the tiger emanating from every pore. Others have it buried deep inside. Where it becomes an extreme challenge to bring it out, **but it's always there**.

Take heart in knowing that you have it, and with development from this book, it may someday save your life.

Society curbs and calms our tiger spirit. It has to. Uncontrolled, it would quickly unravel the fragile fabric that holds together our civilization. Ever since you were a child, you have been taught to subdue outbursts of rage. Any type of violent behavior was quickly stifled, the wildness inside pushed back, so that you could fit in, and be a part of a peaceful society. You have been made civilized. It is not your true nature, but it is necessary, and allows you to get along with the people around you.

The inherent danger of society taming your natural fighting instinct is it will be more difficult to call upon when needed. However, the average goblin doesn't have a problem with viciously attacking you, because he sees you only as an object (not as a human). He has no compassion for you. To him, you are only a target of opportunity. He will have no remorse after hurting or killing you.

You, on the other hand, might hesitate in your counter-attack. This is because we are taught as we grow up to be peaceful and kind to each other. The goblins of the world somehow missed out on that lecture, and will not hesitate to do terrible things to you if you allow them.

One of my best friends, and my first black belt student Mr. Jack Morris recently explained to me how he gets in the way of hesitating in self-defense. At a recent meeting of all of our black belts we had a drunk attempt to start a fight. While I was talking to the trouble maker (who was getting increasingly belligerent), Mr. Morris took up a position to help take the guy out if he tried to attack. Mr. Morris later explained to me that if the drunk had tried to attack he was ready to instantly put him out of commission. He said, "If the drunk had taken a swing, *he* would have made the decision to fight for me, I would no longer have been part of the process. The drunk's hand moving would have been the trigger."

Mr. Morris' concept of the attacker making the decision to fight for you is a great way to overcome hesitation due to compassion. In effect he is saying that there is no other choice but to fight. **To hesitate is not an option.** Hesitating equates death, (which of course is not an acceptable choice). So, when he attacks, he has made the decision for you. There are no ethical or moral considerations to ponder over. He has done all the work for you, and all you will need to do is fight, you can be like a machine.

This chapter intends to **bring your natural tiger instinct to the forefront,** and to teach you to call on it in a controlled manner at will. You will end up with the best of both worlds. You will have the power of a tiger to use in destroying an attacker, while having that power controlled enough to remain civilized.

Think of the nicest, kindest, gentlest person you know. Give me twenty minutes with them, and I can turn them into a tiger. This involves gradually angering the person through insults, and taunting them until they are ready to explode with rage. *At that point they are face-to-face with the tiger inside.*

When this zenith of rage is reached, the body goes through physiological changes that are great for self-defense. The muscles become engorged with oxygen-carrying blood. Powerful pain killers called endorphins are released into the blood stream. They are up to 100 times stronger than morphine. Adrenaline allows the muscles to work at full potential. **The body becomes super-human.**

To the person experiencing this rage, everything seems to go in slow-motion. This is a perception-illusion, caused by their thought process racing at around four times normal speed. In comparison to how fast they are thinking, everything around them seems to have slowed way down. This can help in being able to see oncoming strikes before they hit, giving plenty of time to react.

When this feeling of extreme rage kicks in, **it must be communicated to the dirt-bag.** As Mr. Lee always taught me, "**You must attack all his senses, just as the tiger does.** Communicate to him your severe hatred. Let him see it in your face, let him hear it in your shout, let him feel it from your strike." The visual, the auditory, and the physical blow are all used in conjunction to cause what Mr. Lee would call, *"A stultifying dysfunction between the synapses and the axons."* Or in other words, short circuit his brain and put him in catatonic shock.

When the tiger strikes its prey, it roars with all its might. It shows its teeth and lowers its brow. These actions are not by accident. They are all designed to focus the tiger's complete power toward taking down its prey. Do likewise.

Show your inner rage toward your assailant outwardly by putting on the most hateful look you can. Let him hear your rage by **shouting as loud as you can.** Your shout can be any sound or word you choose. You can yell out a deep guttural sound, or you can shout "die!" or "jerk!" It doesn't matter what is yelled, but it does matter how you do it. It must be the loudest sound you can muster.

Loud sounds have a paralyzing effect on animals, especially when they are unexpected. If a dog or cat runs out in front of your car, the worst thing you can do is honk your horn. The loud unexpected sound of your car's horn makes the dog or cat freeze, resulting in a run-over animal. This paralyzing effect of sound works the same way on people.

Try this experiment. The next time you're talking face-to-face with a friend, try suddenly screaming or yelling at the top of your lungs. Your friend will freeze like a statue for a good two seconds. They will probably think you're crazy, but you will have proven to yourself how effective a strong yell can be in self-defense.

I recall as a teenager being at the San Francisco Zoo's lion and tiger house during feeding time. It was an extremely large room with lion and tiger cages on three sides of the room. I was anxiously awaiting the feeding time for the big cats. As the four o'clock feeding time came around, I found I was the only visitor at the exhibit. Everyone had left. I was soon to find out why.

The big cats knew that food was on the way, and they all started roaring at once in anticipation. There must have been fifteen big cats all roaring at the same time. The sound was deafening. **I suddenly couldn't think.** I knew I wanted to get out, but **I was paralyzed**. I could feel the reverberations of the terrifying roars bouncing off the walls. It took a good ten seconds before I could think straight and move. As soon as my feet allowed, I was out of there.

Since the tiger-exhibit experience, I have always practiced yelling or kiai-ing at full blast while practicing my martial arts technique. It works. Use it. Remember, **attack your assailant on every level possible.**

Let your strike convey intense hatred, and destruction. Compassion and benevolence must temporarily be set aside. He must see death in your eyes. If he feels it strongly enough he will flee, totally abandoning his attack.

Most likely your assailant will not be thinking that you will fight back. He will be attacking you because he will have sensed fear, or weakness. *Surprise him with the tiger.* Your shout combined with the look of death on your face, should be enough to **communicate to him that he has made a grave error, and he'd better run for his life.**

There is a classic urban legend that deals with the tiger spirit. A woman picks up the side of a car to free her trapped child pinned under the tire. This legend is based on actual occurrences. *Powerful, passionate emotions trigger the tiger instinct.*

In the case of the mother and her trapped child, her love for her child was so strong that in order to save her child, the tiger instinct was released, giving her incredible strength to be able to lift the car. My Uncle Terry, a retired police lieutenant, told me of an incident where some nut had run over two pedestrians. One victim ended up trapped under the rear left tire of the car. An officer on the scene, so worried that the person trapped under the car would die, mustered up enough of his tiger instinct to lift that entire side of the car three feet up, freeing the accident victim. The officer's sense of duty, and care for his fellow man was what allowed him to tap into that power.

The super-human strength associated with the tiger instinct can easily be brought out in anyone with the use of the drug P.C.P., commonly called "Angel dust". The drug's effect on the brain is to shut down the otherwise always-active "governor" that limits our body's full potential for strength.

I've had many of my law-enforcement students tell me horror stories associated with trying to control people who are under the influence of P.C.P. The stories are always similar; "It was like trying to wrestle with superman.", or "I hit the guy as hard as I could with my riot baton, and nothing happened, he just kept on fighting." One officer told me of a twelve-year-old boy who punched him during an arrest, and knocked this 200-pound officer seven feet back against his patrol car. He said, "It felt like that kid hit me with a telephone pole."

In another case, my student told me of a car stop where a man under the influence of P.C.P. came at the officer, not stopping when warned to. The officer was forced to fire six rounds into the man, who kept coming like a zombie. The officer reloaded and fired six more rounds; still no response, so he reloaded again, and fired six more rounds. All eighteen rounds were hits. The goblin finally dropped because of a loss of too much blood; otherwise he would of kept on coming.

So does P.C.P. give these people super-human strength? No. **The power is already there.** The drug just shuts down the part of the brain that usually keeps us from being able to do such things. The drug activates the tiger instinct. It also fries the brain, raises the body temperature way beyond normal range, and causes all sorts of other permanent damage. It is a terrible drug that has ruined many lives.

You don't need a drug to bring out your tiger instinct. Remember, **the power is already in you,** all you need is a way to bring it to bear, and to control it. The tool used for this is *emotion.* Through controlling your emotions, you can bring out and use your tiger instinct for defense. Imagine fighting with **five times your normal strength,** being able to take a heavy hit, and not even feel it. **You would be almost invincible.**

Here is the process used to bring out and control the tiger: first you need a catalyst to get your emotions going. This can be done in two different ways. One, you can think back to a time in your life, when, for what ever reason, you were so angry that you could have (or maybe did) drive your fist through a wall. You need only think back to that circumstance to bring the rage back. Or, you can imagine a hypothetical scenario that would drive you to rage.

Typically, what works best is to imagine someone in your family that you love dearly being under attack, and you are the only one who can save their life. Most people use this method. It seems to work best. Remember, you are not being given some sort of magic, mystical powers; instead you are tapping in on a power that you have carried with you since birth.

Most people are familiar with the term "Maternal and Paternal instinct." This is the natural, powerful instinct that a parent has to protect their child. This protective instinct is a great way to tap in on your tiger instinct. I recall hearing on the radio a perfect example of this: A woman was interviewing a martial arts teacher on self-defense concept. She asked, "What do you feel is the most effective way to stop an attacker?" He responded, *"That's easy, you poke out his eyes. If he can't see you, he can't hurt you."*

She was obviously very disturbed by his comment, and replied, " I could never do that." He said, "Even if the guy is going to kill you?" She replied, "No, I couldn't, it's just too gross." Then he tapped in on her natural maternal instinct by asking, "Do you have children?" She said, "Yes, a four-year old daughter." He said, "Imagine the unthinkable, a 250-pound rapist is coming at your daughter, and you are the only thing between him and her. Could you do it then?" She replied without hesitation, *"In a heart beat!"* She was able to picture herself successfully fighting back, when it meant protecting her daughter. **This is the model to copy.**

I am able to instantly go into the tiger mode within one second, simply by thinking of one person. The piece of human garbage who raped my sister. **The mere thought of that dirt-bag instantly makes my blood boil.** Anytime I practice my martial art technique, I think of him. I turn this terrible thought from the past to a positive, giving me super strength which I can use to save my life.

Fear and anger are very closely related emotions. Fear is a natural first-step emotion. What you must learn to do quickly, is to convert fear into anger. *The key is indignation.* You must learn, and practice becoming indignant. **The more unjust the attack, the more angry you must become,** instead of being fearful. Rather than thinking to yourself, "Oh God, there's four of them and one of me, they are going to kill me!" Think instead, "How dare these four punks try and ruin my day! Four against one, that's totally unfair, those low-life scum are going to regret this!" Once again, let the injustice of the attack anger you, instead of scare you. *Become indignant.*

A predator expects its prey to be fearful. *The fear triggers an instinctual green light for the predator to continue the assault.* If no fear is present, the predator will back down.

I used to run three miles between my house and the Kung-Fu school every day. I was too young to drive. Each night on my way home, I would pass a house which had a dog. The dog would chase me for about one block, almost biting me each time. I told my teacher, Mr. Lee, about this. He said, "The dog is only naturally responding to your fear. Tonight on your way home, if the dog approaches you, already have it in your mind that you are the hunter, not the hunted, and that you will destroy the dog if he gets near. *You must feel this in your heart,* because if the dog smells fear he will attack."

Sure enough, that night the dog came running up to me nipping at my heals. I turned around in a fighting stance, and channeled extreme hatred toward the dog. I visualized putting the dog airborne with a snap kick. The dog screeched on his brakes, came to a full stop, and ran in the other direction. **The dog sensed death and wanted no part of it.**

My tiger instinct had been activated by emotion, and the dog could feel it. I like dogs, just as I like people. But neither have the right to hurt me, and with the help of my tiger instinct neither will.

I remember watching a documentary on the Great White Shark that helped me to understand what Mr. Lee had taught me about the tiger instinct. In the documentary an oceanographer was experimenting with the hunting characteristics of the Great White Shark off the Great Barrier Reef of Australia.

He used a remote-controlled video camera to film the sharks during a feeding frenzy. Blood and chum were poured into the ocean to attract the sharks. The first one to arrive was a fifteen-footer. The shark circled the camera twice, and then bumped it to see if it was a viable meal. To get a better look at the shark, the oceanographer moved the camera again, by remote control to pursue the shark. What he noticed surprised and intrigued him. As the camera floated toward the Great White, the shark swam off. **It seemed the shark was not used to it's prey chasing it.**

The oceanographer repeated the experiment with the camera three times to prove his idea. Each time the shark swam off. He then decided to test out his theory with himself as the prospective prey. After attracting another shark with a chum-line, this time a seventeen footer, he entered the open ocean to engage the Great White. The seventeen-footer went into an instinctual hunting pattern of circling the diver. The oceanographer was protected only by a four-foot pole that he kept between him and the shark. The Great White arched it's back, rolled it's eyes back and came in for a bite.

The diver swam at the shark instead of away, and luckily **the shark turned tail, and swam off.** Two minutes later the shark returned and the same scenario was repeated, with the same results. By now, a second Great White swam in and started the same attack pattern.

Each time a shark would approach him, he would swim at the shark, and each time the shark would back off. Finally a third shark showed up, and the oceanographer retreated to his shark cage. He simply could not watch all those predators at once. He proved his theory. *A predator expects a certain prey response, namely fear.* When the opposite occurs and the prey becomes the predator, **the original predator's thinking pattern is short-circuited and the assault is halted.**

This concept works just as well on people as it does on animals. Remember: It's O.K., and normal to have your first response to attack be fear, but you must instantly be able to turn the fear into anger and aggression. *Your assailant does not expect to deal with a tiger.*

When you practice the techniques taught later in the "Stop Button" chapter, **you must activate the tiger.** You need to be accustomed to the increase in adrenaline, and strength. Think of that one thought that brings you to your state of rage, and stay enraged as you strike with all your power. Your heart rate will pick way up, you'll sweat, you may get "tunnel vision", you may feel sick to your stomach. These are all normal reactions that are experienced when the tiger kicks in.

What's important is that you are used to it. Your workout need only last five minutes, but **it should be done often**, so you are used to quickly activating your tiger instinct. When you are finished with your workout, learn to shut it down fast. This is done by breathing very deeply, visualizing your heart slowing down, and by thinking pleasant thoughts. It does take longer to shut down than to start up.

By being proficient with the color code, you'll have a little time to get the tiger instinct fired up while in orange before you need to shift to red. Remember: If the tiger does kick in during orange, you most likely won't need to shift to red. **Because the attacker will feel imminent death,** and back down, just as the dog and shark did.

The only thing that can go wrong with this process is a suicidal response called "self-doubt." **You must practice eliminating self-doubt from every part of your life,** so that it can't raise it's ugly head while you are fighting for your survival. No matter how dire the situation, you must not allow yourself to visualize failure. If you do, it will become a self-fulfilling prophecy. Remember: Change the fear into anger, be indignant. **Become furious** with just the notion of another person trying to hurt you, let alone the act of it.

Mr. Lee used to teach me that self-doubt is like trying to drive with the emergency brake on. "You will get where you are going, but it takes you a lot longer, and you use a lot more energy in the process." Only visualize victory. It is surprisingly physically easy to take out an assailant; the only thing that will prevent you is not applying your full strength because of self-doubt.

What price do you pay by not fighting back? You will for sure lose your dignity, and self-respect. You may sustain a permanent, crippling injury. *You may lose your most prized possession, your life.* You will empower your attacker to commit many more assaults. You will break the heart of all the people who care about you, whose lives will be permanently changed for the worse, because you are gone. **This is the price of not fighting back.**

Some people say that when attacked, do what ever the fiend wants, and he'll probably not hurt you. If raped, just go along with it, don't struggle. Give the robber what ever he wants. Don't resist, or do anything to make the attacker angry, just obey the psycho's commands.

These are fitting comments for the unprepared, for what other choice do they have? They don't know how to fight back, so they feel that they are at the mercy of the assailant.

You on the other hand are much different, because after reading and taking to heart the preceding chapters, you will be mentally prepared to fight. Because of your knowledge of the Color Code, you will not have been surprised, and after practicing the techniques taught in the next chapter, you will be physically prepared to go to battle. **You have a choice!**

If you have no means to defend yourself, you are at the mercy of the attacker. People who think along these lines don't like books like this one, nor do they enjoy listening to the evening news. They don't want to think of attack, they want to pretend they have an ***"exempt sticker"*** on their forehead, and are immune from attack. They want to deny and hide their head in the sand. Rather than prepare, they make the fatal error of thinking their attacker will either be too compassionate, or too fearful of legal implications to hurt them. Their ineptitude and sheer lack of dignity has permitted violent crime and mass murderers to terrorize our society for centuries.

Their entire premise of non-action is flawed. What kind of individual goes around committing violent crime? A truthful, compassionate, law-abiding citizen? Of course not, but these poor people are willing to sheepishly do whatever the psycho wants, hoping he'll have mercy on them. They think that goblins think the way they do. Fat chance! Goblins are sub-human vermin that understand only one thing, terror. They understand how to inflict it, and **they back away from it when it's focused against them.**

In the tiger mode you bring terror to your assailant. Your terror-infliction against the assailant must be even more vicious than his. Your rage focused on your opponent must surpass even his worst nightmare. In essence, **you must temporarily become more psychotic than your assailant**. It is the only thing he'll understand.

Like most people, I would prefer a world where pacifism works. But until such a peaceful world exists, you need to waken, develop, and rely on the tiger within.

Quotes from the "Stop Button" Chapter

"No matter how intent your assailant is on hurting you, *he will not even think of you after you strike his eyes.* His total attention will shift to himself. He will grab his face, screaming with the fear that he is blinded forever."
PAGE 34

"I always teach my younger students to think of the eyes as two big **"Stop buttons."** I tell them that if a stranger is trying to hurt them, they must press those stop buttons. Use this same simple mind set. Visualize two big stop buttons. *They are your primary targets."*
PAGE 34

"Striking first will have such a shocking effect on your assailant that he won't be able to stop your strike, and if your initial strike is to a function target the fight will be over, most likely in *under one second."*
PAGE 36

"THE CIRCLE OF FEAR:　This is an imaginary line at six feet in any direction around you. The circle of fear represents the line that when crossed by your assailant forces you into action. The survivor of the conflict will be *the one who strikes first.* Make sure that's you."
PAGE 36

"Blocking is a fool's game.　If your assailant is a proficient fighter, and you are waiting for him to hit first, you probably won't get the chance to respond. By the time your brain registers　that you need to block, he will already have made contact."
PAGE 39

CHAPTER FOUR

THE "STOP BUTTON"

Your ability to defend yourself is ninety percent your mental set, and ten percent your physical technique. This chapter will teach you a few extremely effective techniques designed **to end the fight within one second.** My teacher would always say, " **If the fight lasts more than three seconds you are playing a game, and a deadly game at that."** Every second the fight is allowed to continue, your chances of coming out of it unscathed rapidly diminish. Your element of surprise wears off, your assailant has time to find a weakness in your defense, and if you are dealing with multiple goblins, your delay allows them to surround you. Remember, your strategy is to do everything in your power to avoid the fight, but if it must happen *you need to explode with rage, and end the fight in one second.*

The major key in successful use of martial art strikes is where they are directed. You must become a **"Head hunter."** Your number-one target must always be the head. If a bomb went off in the room next to you, I can guarantee that the first thing you would do is cover your head with both arms. You wouldn't cover your knee, or your chest, or your butt. You would instinctively cover your control center, your head. Because *you are your head.* You can get along without your arm, and without your leg, even without some of your torso, but you cannot make it without your head. The body should only be hit in preparation to attacking the head.

There are two main categories of targets on the human body--**pain, and function.** Pain targets, when hit, disable the attacker by causing enough pain to distract the opponent's attention away from hurting you. Function targets are areas of the body that when struck destroy or weaken a function such as vision, breathing, circulation, or locomotion.

Our main focus will be on **function targets,** as pain targets rely on our assailant being able to experience pain, which is often not the case. Calm, sane, rational people do not go around attacking others. Drugged up, and/or psychotic people are the ones to worry about. They most often don't feel pain. Either they are so psychotic that their endorphins are kicked in, blocking pain sensation, or they are numb from alcohol and drugs.

Hitting pain targets is a gamble, and *you shouldn't gamble with your life.* Pain targets should only be chosen when **function** targets are not available.

The main function target, causing the most traumatic result when hit, is the eyes. Our **vision is eighty percent of our perception of the world.** When that is taken away, the fight immediately stops. Also, **your assailant can't hit what he can't see.** If your assailant can feel pain, and you hit his eyes, you will have dealt him the most painful blow possible.

It's important to prove this to yourself, because *you won't use what you don't believe in.* Try this. Press in on some of the function targets mentioned earlier. Press your index finger against your temple. That should hurt a little. Now, press your finger in against your windpipe, just below the adam's apple. That should feel very uncomfortable, and may cause you to cough. Next, hold open your right eye with your left hand, as you take your right index finger, and press in on your exposed eyeball. Well, if you were able to touch the eyeball, you can now understand how painful an attack on the eyes would be.

As an experiment, for one year I would ask beginning students on their first lesson where they felt the best place was to hit an assailant to instantly stop the attack. What I heard most often was, "I would kick 'em in the groin." Or, "I'd punch him in the gut." None of the hundreds of people I asked said they would poke out the eyes. I asked my teacher why people have such a hard time with the idea of striking the eyes. He said, "People don't want to do to their attacker what they feel will be done back to them." However, logic tells us that if we poke out an attacker's eyes there is no way he can do the same to us, because he won't be able to see us.

The anxiety associated with striking an assailant's eyes probably goes back to grade school, when playground fights were basically one kid copying the attack of the other kid. Little Billy punches you in the shoulder, so you punch little Billy back on the shoulder. Then he puts you in a headlock. So, then you put him in a headlock, etc., etc. I've even seen grown men fighting this way, where one guy copies the attack of the guy who hits him. The reality is, if you strike your assailant's eyes, he will be out of commission for a long time. **He will not be able to return the attack.**

As a young man I quickly learned how effective an eye strike can be. To help pay for my martial arts lessons, I got a paper route. The last part of my route was at the end of a long, steep street called Potrero. Each day after my final delivery, I would zoom down Potrero on my bike headed for home. One day I was trying to see how fast I could race down the street. I had just installed a speedometer on my bike, and being young and foolish I brought my speed up to sixty m.p.h. My eyes were watering, the front wheel was wobbling, and just as I was about to put on the brakes, I drove through a swarm of gnats. Four or five hit my eyes. **At sixty m.p.h., I let go of the handle bars with both hands and grabbed my face!**

You can probably imagine what happened next. I woke up about twelve feet from where my bike lay in a mangled heap. I was covered with blood, and had lost a lot of skin. I was picking small pieces of gnats out of my eyes for the next two days. The moral of the story is, there is no way I would ever do that again. If I were offered ten million dollars, or even one hundred million dollars to let go of my bikes handle bars with both hands at sixty m.p.h., I wouldn't do it. What good is one hundred million dollars to me if I'm dead? It would be suicide to do that again.

The point is, the pain of those gnats hitting my eyes was so severe that **all logical thinking went out the window,** and I just couldn't help but grab my face. The pain was that severe.

No matter how intent your assailant is on hurting you, **he will not even think of you after you strike his eyes.** His total attention will shift to himself. He will grab his face, screaming with the fear that he is blinded forever. Remember, you will have taken away eighty percent of his senses with your one strike. **No other martial arts strike is as devastating.**

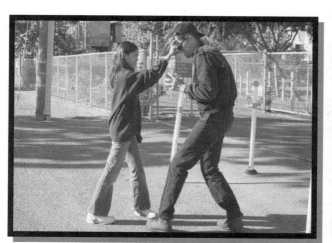
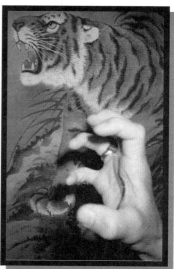

USE A TIGER'S CLAW TO GET PAST GLASSES.

I always teach my younger students to think of the eyes as two big **"Stop buttons."** I tell them that if a stranger is trying to hurt them, they must press those stop buttons. Use this same simple mind set. Visualize two big stop buttons. **They are your primary targets.**

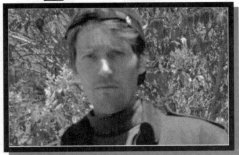

HOW THE GOBLIN WANTS YOU TO SEE HIM.

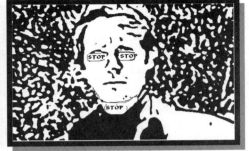

YOU SHOULD SEE ONLY TARGETS.

If the eyes are not available, target number two is the wind-pipe. With four pounds or more of pressure per square inch impact directed below the adam's apple, you will be able to crush this cartilage-formed pipe, closing it off. Your assailant will immediately start to gag, he will grab for his throat with both hands. If his wind-pipe is not surgically opened up within three minutes, he will die. You are only allowed to strike this target when it can be proved the goblin had the ability and the intent to kill you. Remember, don't hesitate! If you feel your life is threatened, don't take the time to consider why. **React, save your life.**

The temple, along with the jugular vein/carotid-artery complex, are your number three targets. They are not picked first because they are not as dependable for stopping attackers. I've struck sparring opponents in the temple where they have gone unconscious on impact, and I've seen people go unconscious when their blood supply to the brain was cut off. So I know these targets are effective, but they do take energy and skill to damage.

For most people, a blow of eight pounds per square inch directed at the temple is enough to cause a "knock out." But some must have thicker skulls because it takes more power to cause the same effect. A powerful chop directed at the side of the neck is normally enough to cause the carotid artery/jugular vein complex to be obstructed, and to cause a "knock out," but it takes a fair amount of skill to make this strike effective.

Once again, be a head hunter, **go for the eyes first.** Second, the wind-pipe, and third--the temple or the carotid artery.

Be prepared to hit numerous times. Your goal is to end the fight with one hit, but consider what type of person you will be fighting. Most likely you will encounter a zombie-like assailant impervious to pain. He's probably very accustomed to getting hit. He most likely has led a violent life, full of fights, being struck on almost a daily basis. Your one hit might not be enough. Have it in your head that you will keep hitting until he is no longer a threat.

YOU MUST HIT FIRST!!!! This goes against most people's self-defense beliefs. The majority of people have been conditioned to not strike unless hit first. This is a nice "touchy-feely" type concept, but it's apt to get you killed. Allowing your assailant the first blow goes exactly along with his plan. **You striking first will give you a considerable advantage,** and remember you are morally and legally justified in doing so as long as the goblin has the present ability and intent to cause you great bodily harm or death. **Beat him to it.**

Striking first will have such a shocking effect on your assailant that he won't be able to stop your strike, and if your initial strike is to a function target the fight will be over, most likely in **under one second.**

THE CIRCLE OF FEAR: This is an imaginary line at six feet in any direction around you. The circle of fear represents the line that when crossed by your assailant forces you into action. The survivor of the conflict will **be the one who strikes first.** Make sure that's you. Here are some examples of how to strike from within the circle:

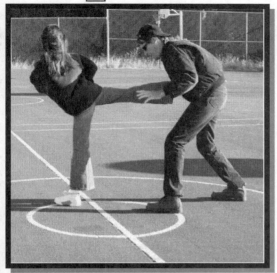

*USE A REAR KICK IF HE
ATTACKS FROM BEHIND.*

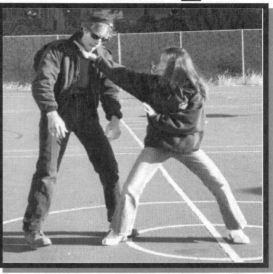

*USE A QUICK CHOP IF HE
ATTACKS FROM THE SIDE.*

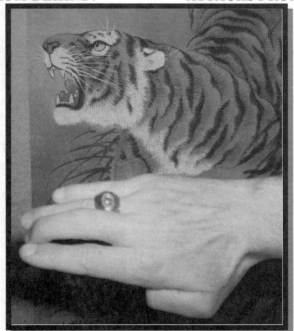

PROPER HAND POSITION FOR A CHOP.

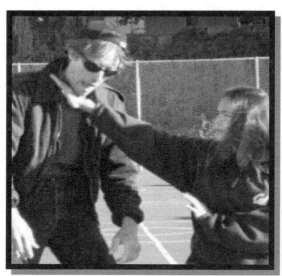

*JUST FOUR POUNDS OF
PRESSURE WILL STOP HIM.*

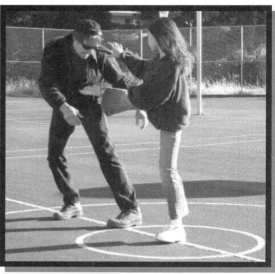

*USE YOUR FEET AS A FIRST
STRIKE WEAPON.*

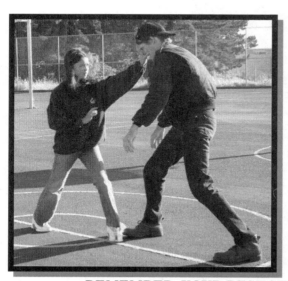

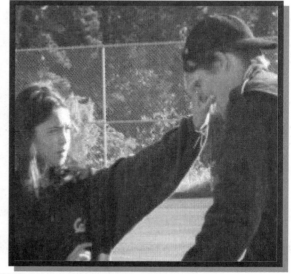

*REMEMBER, YOUR BEST STRIKE IS ALWAYS AN ATTACK ON
THE EYES. "IF HE CAN'T SEE YOU, HE CAN'T HURT YOU."*

Blocking is a fool's game. If your assailant is a proficient fighter, and you are waiting for him to hit first, you probably won't get the chance to respond. By the time your brain registers that you need to block, he will already have made contact. You have, at best, if you are lucky, a twenty percent chance of being able to block his strike. That means there is an eighty percent chance of getting hit. So, when blocking, your life is hanging on the hope that your attacker is slow, and that you are lucky. This is far too great of a gamble. Remember the bazooka concept. You do everything to avoid the fight, but if there is no way out, **strike first, strike hard, and go for function, not pain.**

It's crucial that you believe in the first-strike strategy. Here is a little experiment that I think will prove it to you. Stand two feet away from a friend. If you are right handed, have your right shoulder toward your friend, visa versa if you are left handed. Tell him or her that you are going to tap their shoulder, and that you want him or her to knock away your hand before you are able to tap the shoulder. Do it slowly, then medium speed, to make sure your friend gets the feel of how to knock away your hand. Then tell him or her that you are going to go full speed.

It's important that you both start this drill with both hands at your sides. Next go full speed, tap the shoulder and snap your hand back as fast as you can. If your friend is lucky, he or she might have been able to knock your hand (on it's way back). **Had you been striking the eye, instead of tapping the shoulder, you would have had his or her eye in your hand.**

Try this drill on a few friends, not just your slow friends. You do have to try to go full speed to make this work. I've done this drill on over two hundred people and it's worked every time, without exception.

By now you should be a firm believer in striking first. Consider this: You warned your friend what you were about to do, you then had them practice blocking your strike, and you still got them, before they got you. Imagine how well this will work on the goblin **who doesn't even think you are going to fight back, let alone strike first.**

When dealing with a multiple dirt-bag attack, striking first will most certainly save your life. If you wait for one creep to hit, you will surely be overrun. By the time you counter attack (if you're able), the other goblins will be all over you.

I want you to survive! Don't fight fair, fight to win. Get it ingrained in your head now that if attacked, **you will strike first.** When you practice your awareness training, doing imaginary shifts between code yellow and code orange, visualize the response you put together in orange, as **you hitting first.** This will change the many years of opposite programming you have been hit with since being a toddler. "Don't hit first, fight fair" has been pounded in your brain, since you were a kid. It may have been a good idea back when you were knee high to a grass-hopper, but it is now very dangerous baggage that could get you killed.

If you are caught totally unaware, and your attacker is able to grab you, you will be in extreme danger. The following are simple techniques to get out of grabs. If a psycho grabs one of your arms, **don't play his game** (strength vs. strength), instead fight smart. Take your free hand and destroy either his eyes, his throat, or his temple. If he's dumb enough to grab you with both hands on your one arm, once again, use your free hand **to hit his eyes!**

If he is in front of you grabbing your neck, shoulders, or waist, take your free hand (or hands) and **go for the eyes.** If you are grabbed in such a way where your hands are out of commission, u**se your feet.** Look for one of his feet, and destroy it. Drive your heel down on the meatiest part of his foot. Make sure to rake down his shin on your way down to crushing his foot.

DEFENSE AGAINST A GRAB WITH ARMS PINNED

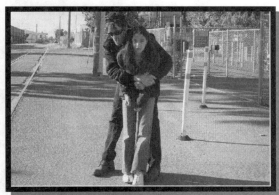

VICTIM CAN'T USE HER HANDS TO FIGHT

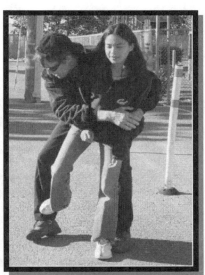

SHE IMMEDIATELY USES HER FEET TO ATTACK

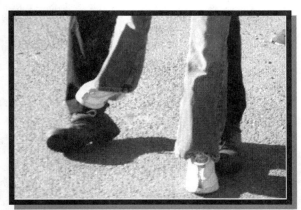

THE FINAL STRIKE IS TO STOMP DOWN ON THE MEATY PART OF THE FOOT OR ANKLE.

STOPPING A CHOKE FROM THE FRONT

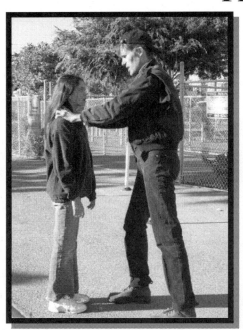

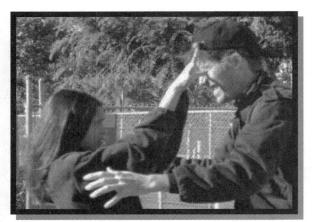

A CHOICE ATTACK IS VERY DANGEROUS AND
SHOULD BE COUNTERED BY A QUICK BLINDING TECHNIQUE.

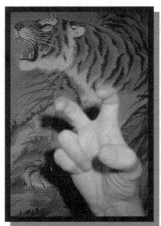

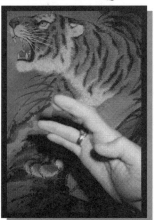

**The Falcon's talon, also known
as two dragons fighting for the pearl.**

The rigid claw.

DEFENSE AGAINST A CHOKE
FROM BEHIND

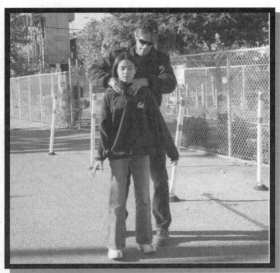

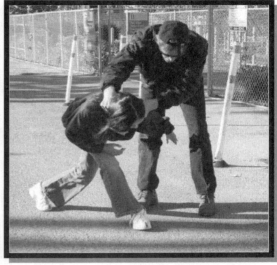

IT ONLY TAKES ONE SECOND FOR THE
ATTACKER TO CAUSE FATAL DAMAGE.

STEP BEHIND YOUR OWN LEG AS YOU
BEND FORWARD AND CHOP HIS GROIN.

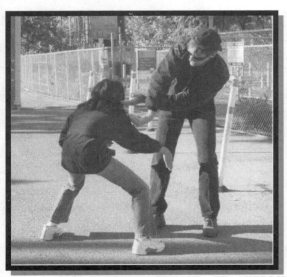

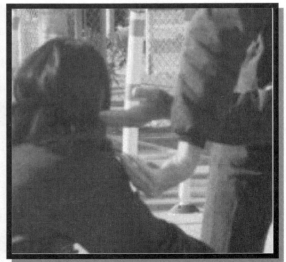

**TURN UNDERNEATH YOUR ATTACKERS HANDS AS YOU STRIKE THE GROIN AGAIN
WITH THE RIDGE OF YOUR HAND. WHAT SAVES YOUR LIFE IS GOING BELOW YOUR
ATTACKERS GRIP. EVEN A VERY POWERFUL PERSON WON'T BE ABLE TO HOLD YOU.**

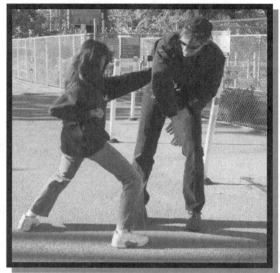

FOLLOW UP WITH A QUICK PUNCH TO THE
BODY.

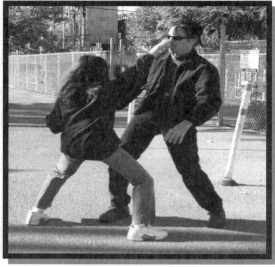

FOCUS YOUR LAST FULL POWER
STRIKE TO THE HEAD.

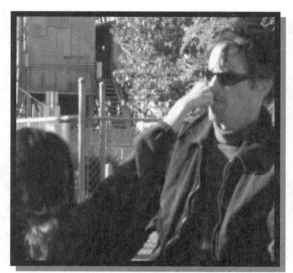

REMEMBER, THE HEAD IS ALWAYS THE
PRIMARY TARGET.

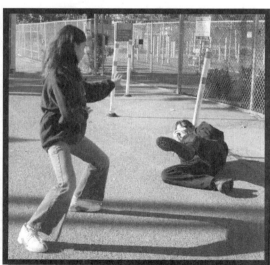

ALWAYS GAIN DISTANCE FROM
THE ATTACKER AS SOON AS POSSIBLE.

Biting can be an effective weapon. Almost all animals will bite when provoked. **Do the same, it works!!** If some jerk puts his hand over your mouth to keep you from screaming, make *him* scream by biting off one of his fingers.

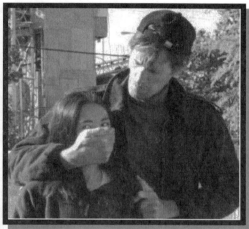

IF SOMEONE COVERS YOUR MOUTH-- BITE AS HARD AS YOU CAN.

During a rape, often the proposed victim ends up lying on the ground, face up with their arms somehow pinned. For the sexual assault to go forward, the psycho must partially disrobe himself, and the proposed victim. This is a big-time error on the part of the dirt-bag, which **you must not allow him to recover from.** The millisecond the creep goes to disrobe himself or you, he will have to release one of your hands. Like a rocket, **drive your free hand into his eye,** spring to your feet while he is blinded, strike again if needed and then get out of there. If the rapist goes to kiss your mouth, bite his lip until your teeth meet. As his hands go to save his torn lip, once again at least one of your hands will be free. **Remember: poke his eyes, get up and run.**

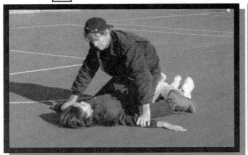

IF PINNED ON THE GROUND

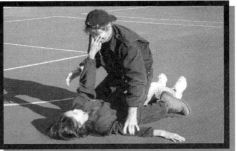

STRIKE THE EYES TO BREAK FREE.

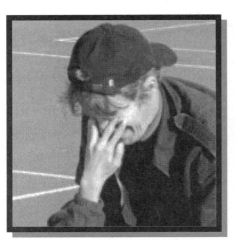

JAB HIS EYES WITH YOUR FREE HAND

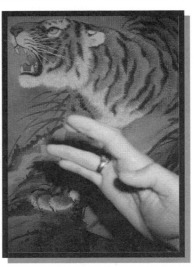

THE WEAPON USED IS A RIGID CLAW.

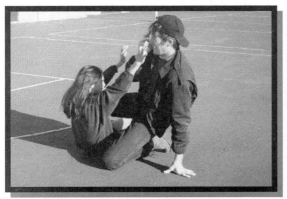

*USE BOTH HANDS TO PUSH AT
THE FACE.*

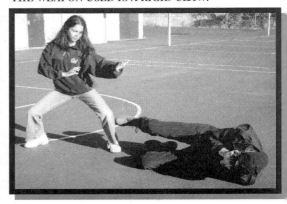

*QUICKLY PUT DISTANCE BETWEEN
YOU AND THE ASSAILANT.*

As you can see from this chapter, the physical technique necessary to stop an attack is fairly easy. It is important to physically practice these strikes often. Many students have bought styrofoam wig heads for a couple of bucks to practice hitting the head. This is especially effective for developing the accuracy needed to attack the eyes.

If you have studied the preceding chapters thoroughly, you will be mentally prepared for battle, and you will be aware enough not to be caught off guard. With the simple strikes taught in this chapter, **you will be able to stop the fight in one second.**

Quotes from
Home Defense Chapter

"Polly Klass was kidnapped from her home while everyone was awake. Her mother never knew that a stranger had entered her home. Unfortunately, their house was not set up well as a deterrent. Let's learn from her tragedy, so that it won't be repeated."
PAGE 55

"Keep a powerful flashlight near the head of your bed. A four or six-cell **large metal** flashlight is highly recommended. After blinding your assailant with the powerful beam of the flashlight, you can **then club the goblin over the head with it."**
PAGE 56

"Having a dog, an alarm system, good lighting, and good visibility are all good deterrents by themselves. Why not put them all together and **make your home the one that never gets picked?"**
PAGE 57

"If you don't fight back, you may get lucky and be one of the minority who are only raped and terrorized, but not killed. The odds are in your favor if you fight. Your chance of survival goes way up, and **you become the one in control,** instead of the goblin."
PAGE 59

"It's very important to fight back right at the onset of trouble. The longer you wait to fight back, the more paralyzed you become with fear. **When you wait, you effectively come under the spell of your assailant."**
PAGE 60

"Dirt-bags know that home owners leave their windows open in hot weather, and purposefully **pick hot days to commit their evil deeds."**
PAGE 62

CHAPTER FIVE

Home Defense

Your home or dwelling should be the one place where you can really feel safe and secure. After coming home from a long day at work, you should be able to relax, without the worry of attack. For the most part you can relax as long as you have taken a few preventative measures, and you continue to live by the awareness concepts taught earlier in this book.

Your home is an extension of yourself. Since you are the type of person who is prepared to deal with self-defense this should also be true of your house, and since your home is your sanctuary *an attack on it should infuriate you just as much as a direct attack on yourself.*

Just as with a personal attack, the number one thing to be concerned with is **prevention.** You must become an expert in making your home extremely uninviting to goblins. Remember, dirt-bags who attempt robberies or home invasions want it easy. They are lazy, opportunistic low-lifes. If your house seems to be the easiest house on your block to break into, guess what? You are going to have a problem.

The following simple, common sense steps will make your house the one that never gets picked.

KEYS: Always have your house key in hand as you approach your front door. Many people have fallen victim to home-invaders while scrambling for their keys at the last minute. Remember, **attackers love to find victims that are distracted.** Have your key ready to go so you can make a fast entry.

DOGS: Your best bet for keeping away goblins is to either have (or make them think you have) a dog. This has been proven in crime study after crime study. **Dirt-bags are deathly afraid of dogs.** A dog's sense of smell is many hundreds of times stronger than ours. They can smell and/or hear an intruder long before we can.

The dog is not only a great deterrent, but also a very sensitive alarm system. To purchase a system with proximity sensors and detectors to rival the sensitivity of a dog would cost thousands of dollars. When your dog senses an intruder, you find out about it instantly. Your dog barks loudly, becomes very agitated and runs around wildly until the threat subsides. Plus that barking, growling, and running around is enough to send almost any dirt-bag running.

For various reasons some people are unable to keep a dog. This could be due to an allergic reaction, not having sufficient room, or it could be because of the expense of keeping and caring for a dog. Even if you can't have a real dog you can make a would-be intruder **think you have a dog,** which ultimately is just as good.

For three or four dollars you can buy an extra-large dog food bowl, to place in a very visible place outside your house. I recommended you write with a marker across the front of the bowl, the name,**"KILLER"**, or **"BONE CRUSHER"**, etc. (Use your imagination). For a couple of dollars you should buy the biggest **BEWARE OF DOG** signs you can find. At least two. One for the front, and one for the back of the house. Make sure to post them where a goblin casing your house would see them. While you're at it, why not post up a **NO SOLICITORS** sign? All this can be purchased for around ten dollars.

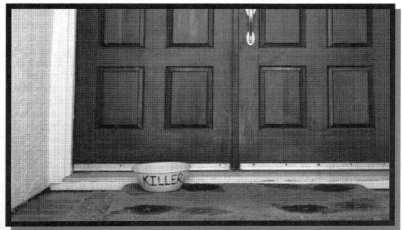

A LARGE DOG FOOD BOWL WITH THE NAME "KILLER" IS A GOOD DETERRENT.

If you would like to spend a little more, (and you enjoy James Bond style electronic gadgets), I recommend you purchase an "Electronic dog." This is simply a small box that plugs into an electrical outlet, which when activated by noise, emits the sound of a very large dog barking. You can purchase this on the internet at many great self-defense product sites. The price is very reasonable for the protection this devise gives you. You can use your internet search engine to find a good site. Just type in the key words: **self-defense products.**

Having a trained attack dog is a nice luxury, but not necessary. Even a little chihuahua will be able to warn you of an intruder long before he gets into your house, and bad guys are usually **afraid of all dogs,** regardless of the dog's size. Another benefit of having a dog for defense is: when you have your dog with you outside your home, you once again have an excellent deterrent to keep low-lifes away from you.

ALARM SYSTEMS: A highly-visible alarm system is an excellent deterrent to would-be home invaders. The trick is to make your system **highly visible.** You can spend as little as $20.00, or you can spend a small fortune on a system. It's up to you. Most home-insurance carriers will give you as much as a 20% decrease on your home policy if you have an alarm system installed. Here are the basics to keep in mind for a home alarm system:

Number one, you want everyone who comes near your house to **know you have an alarm.** Secondly you need some system in place to wake you up should someone enter your home while you're asleep. Beyond these basics, there are a multitude of extra features that you can tie into a system.

One inexpensive method is to purchase an alarm bell box that mounts on the outside of your house. You can find these for as little as $15.00 at many electronic parts stores, and at some locksmiths. The bell box is simply a metal box about 20" high by 20" wide by 8" deep. You can nail, or screw the box onto the front of your house in a very conspicuous place.

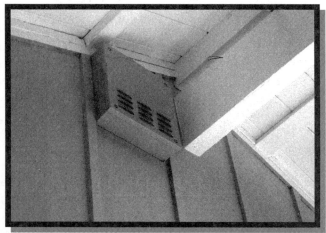

ALARM BOX SCARES AWAY BURGLARS AND HOME INVADERS.

For a few dollars more you can purchase stickers to place on your alarm box, your front and back doors, as well as your windows. The stickers read: **THIS HOUSE IS ELECTRONICALLY PROTECTED.** Even though it really isn't, the dirt-bag will think it is, and instead go after a home without stickers. Remember, goblins don't want a challenge, and because there are countless thousands of unprotected homes in your same neighborhood they will go after them instead. **For a few dollars, you will have saved yourself untold anguish, and maybe even from being killed by a home invader.**

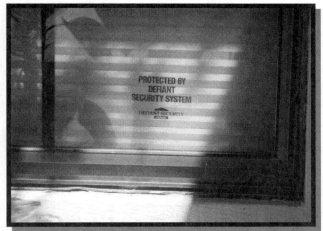

PUT WARNING STICKERS ON ALL WINDOWS AND DOORS.

You must also have a system in place to wake you up if someone enters the area where you sleep. **When you're deep asleep, you are most vulnerable to being attacked.** Unless you have an early warning system in place to wake you up, you will be at the mercy of your attacker. Your only chance of survival will be if your assailant is incompetent and doesn't kill you with his first blow.

So, how can you set up your bedroom to wake you up if someone enters? You can buy an inexpensive motion detector. I've seen them for $10.00. They are usually battery-powered. You set it on your night-stand or dresser, aimed at the entry door to your room. The second a person enters, the detector emits an ear-piercing siren that would wake the dead. If you want to go cheaper you can buy a couple of cow-bells to put on the door handle, so when the door is opened it clangs, waking you up. You can put tin cans filled with little rocks on your windows, so when opened the cans fall and startle you awake.

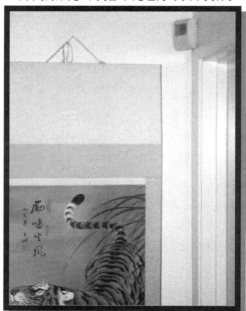

MOTION DETECTOR POSITIONED OUTSIDE OF BEDROOM

There are many systems available for between two and three hundred dollars that are very effective, and easy to install. I recommend the type that uses wireless transmitters, because they are a lot easier to install than the conventional type which involves wires running everywhere.

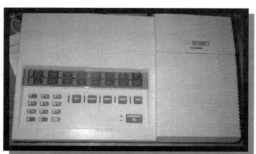

TYPICAL $200.00 WIRELESS ALARM SYSTEM

If you do buy and set up one of these more elaborate systems, make sure to have it on while you're home.

Polly Klass was kidnapped from her home while everyone was awake. Her mother never knew that a stranger had entered her home. Unfortunately, their house was not set up well as a deterrent. Let's learn from her tragedy, so that it won't be repeated.

LIGHTS: Home invaders, being the evil vermin that they are, prefer the darkness. It is in your best interest to spend a few dollars and buy some flood-lights with motion detectors. I've seen these for as little as $10.00 at home improvement stores. They do take a little electrical know-how to set up. If it's beyond your scope, ask a friend who's got the knowledge to help you out. It's a bit of a hassle, but it's worth it. Flood-light motion detectors are very effective deterrents; **I advise having at least two.** One for the front of the property, and one for the back. One on each side of the house as well would be ideal.

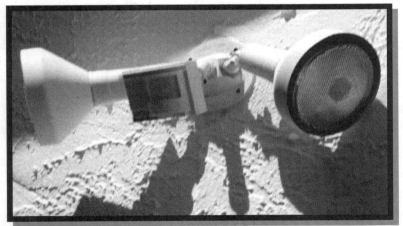

MOTION DETECTING FLOOD LIGHTS FOR OUTSIDE YOUR HOUSE.

It's a great idea to leave on at least one light somewhere in the house while you're sleeping. A would-be invader will think that someone is still awake, and will not pursue their attack. Many people use five dollar timers to automatically turn on a light at night-fall. You can also buy an inexpensive photo-sensor that activates your light when darkness falls. Having an automatic light is crucial when you're away on vacation. Also, a news-talk program playing on your radio can fool an intruder into thinking that you're home.

It is important that you know your home's floor plan so well that you can navigate it in near complete darkness. This is a tremendous advantage you'll have over the home invader who attacks in the dark. Keep a powerful flashlight near the head of your bed. A four or six-cell metal type flashlight is highly recommended. After blinding your assailant with the powerful beam of the flashlight, you can **then club the goblin over the head with it.** The flashlight makes a nice, heavy metal club. Most hardware stores carry this type of flashlight

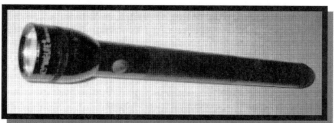

YOU SHOULD CARRY A LARGE METAL FLASHLIGHT IN YOUR CAR AND HAVE ONE IN YOUR BEDROOM FOR USE AS A STRONG LIGHT AND AS A WEAPON.

VISIBILITY: Keep vegetation around your home cut down, especially near windows. You don't want to have an area where a dirt-bag can be out of sight of the neighbors while he is breaking into your home. Keep your blinds or drapes closed, especially at night. You don't want a would-be intruder to know if you are the only one home. At night, with your drapes open and lights on, **you are well-lit and very visible to someone outside your window.** However, someone outside your window is nearly invisible to you.

Devise a way for you to see who's at your door, without the person outside being able to see you. Probably the best way to do this is to install a door-viewer. The door-viewer allows you to see out, but the person outside can't see in. I recommend an extra large door-viewer, that gives you the full view of your front area. Looking out your window to see who's at the door is not a good idea, unless you happen to be a very large, menacing-looking person-- **otherwise, don't let them see you.**

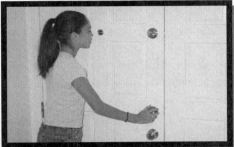 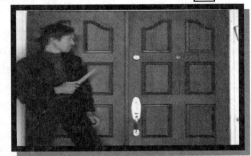

ALWAYS CHECK WHO'S THERE BEFORE OPENING YOUR DOOR.
IF YOU CAN'T SEE WHO'S THERE, DON'T OPEN THE DOOR.

If you currently don't have a way to see who is at your door, your options are: **Install a door viewer right away,** or don't ever answer the door. I can't tell you how many people have been hurt or killed by psychos whose victims simply let them in, never knowing who was at the door.

Having a dog, an alarm system, good lighting, and good visibility are all good deterrents by themselves. Why not put them all together and **make your home the one that never gets picked?** Most of the devices mentioned in this chapter are available online at many great web-sites for self-defense products. Use your search engine and check under: **self-defense products.**

Even with all the best preventative measures in place, there's still no guarantee that you and your home will not some day be threatened. If it does happen, **remember to become indignant.** You must be extremely angry that some low-life has come to your place of refuge to disrupt your tranquility. *Don't be afraid, be angry.*

If someone you don't know enters your home, the law allows you to assume that they are there to cause you great bodily harm, or death. You will not be required to prove it. *You are allowed to take what ever action is necessary to ensure your safety, even to the point of killing the intruder.* As is true with personal self-defense, if you can escape the whole situation without needing to fight, you should do so. Get to your neighbor's house and call the police. It's the job of the police to deal with such problems. However, if there is someone in your house who's in danger of being hurt by the intruder, you need to stay and **take care of business.** By the time it takes the police to arrive, it will be too late.

When you arrive home, if you notice something that makes you think that an intruder is in your home **don't go in.** You might suspect someone is in your home because you notice an unfamiliar car in your driveway, you see someone moving around or notice signs of a break-in, like your door has been kicked in, or a broken window. Whatever the reason, **don't go in.** The only exception would be if a family member is in trouble. Otherwise, go to a neighbor and call the police.

ANSWERING THE DOOR: Every person in your home must be taught the correct procedure for answering the door. Hundreds of people each year are terrorized or **killed by psychos who simply walk in the front door.**

Here is the procedure that you and your family must have as second nature. It must be followed to the letter. **Many goblins are experts at tricking their victims into letting them enter the house.**

Number one, **you must be able to see who is at your door.** A familiar voice is not enough. One particular dirt-bag, responsible for 26 rapes over a two-month period, gained access to his victim's dwellings by meowing like a cat, while scratching at the door. When these unfortunate women would open the door to let in the nice little kitty, they got much more than they had bargained for.

Number two, **never open your door to a stranger.** The only exception would be to let in a person that you are expecting. For example, a repair person, but still only after they have shown their identification through the door-viewer. If you have an uneasy feeling about the repairman, tell him you need to cancel, call the company and ask for them to send someone else. Don't feel ashamed or embarrassed by not letting the person in. **If your gut feeling is that he is trouble, he probably is.** After letting him in, it's too late.

Even if the person at your door looks official, for example he looks like a police officer, fireman or city official, once again **don't let him in,** unless he shows you proper I.D. Don't feel bad about calling the department he represents to verify his identity before letting him in. I have studied many accounts of home attacks perpetrated by psychos impersonating emergency personnel. **Don't be fooled.**

Another common ruse used by home invaders is to work as a team to trick their victims into letting them in. Often a man and woman work together to gain access to you and your home. In one particular example, a woman came banging on the door of the victim, yelling and screaming,"He's going to kill me, he's already raped me, you've got to let me in! I see him, he's only three houses away! You've got to open this door, he'll kill me!" Well, the kind woman did open the door, and for her kindness she and her family paid the ultimate price.

As soon as she opened the door, the Bonnie and Clyde duo both entered, and after finding out where all the valuables where they shot and killed everyone in the house. So, what should you do in a similar situation? **Don't open the door! Call 911** and get the police there as quickly as possible.

Remember, you've got to teach your family these rules. If just one of them blows it, you will all be in danger. You might feel that all this sounds harsh or overly cautious. But, it's better to be cautious than dead.

If everything goes wrong and you end up with some psycho in your home giving you commands with the threat of violence, **do not obey him.** You may feel that if you cooperate, you won't get hurt. *WRONG!!!* Recent crime studies show that the majority of the time the home invader kills his victim after getting what he wants. The reason is either to get rid of the witnesses, or just plain evil.

In another example, two older teens broke into a woman's house, terrorizing her for hours. After raping her repeatedly and forcing her to tell where her jewelry, credit cards and cash were, they took turns kicking her in the stomach. She survived to give police their description, but the seven-month old infant in her womb did not. Obviously the maniacs who attacked her knew that she was pregnant, and purposefully kicked her in the stomach out of pure evil.

If you don't fight back you may get lucky and be one of the minority who are only raped and terrorized, but not killed. The odds are in your favor if you fight. Your chance of survival goes way up, and **you become the one in control,** instead of the goblin.

Whenever you defy the command of a psycho (especially an armed nut-case) you temporarily **short-circuit his thinking process,** giving you two to three seconds to either escape, or attack. If you choose to attack, remember: **go for a function target, in particular, the eyes.** I often hear people say, "Sure, I'll fight back, but what if he has a gun?" You actually have a very good chance of overwhelming your attacker, even if he is armed with a gun.

Most often an armed attacker only has the gun there as an instrument of terror. **He is not prepared to use it.** More times than not, the gun is not even loaded, or it's a toy gun. Dirt-bags feel that if caught by the police with a fake or unloaded gun they will get in less trouble.

Many times the vermin who are willing to use a gun to intimidate are too stupid to know how to properly load and fire a handgun. When an armed assailant gives you the command, **"LAY DOWN!",** and instead of sheepishly laying down you knock the gun to the side and jab your fingers into his eyes, he's going to be very confused. He'll be thinking, "Hey, I said lay down", and the next thing he knows the lights are out. You may not only have saved your life, but also the other people in your home with you. Not to mention the other victims he may have killed in the future had you not taken action, and stopped him.

It's very important to fight back right at the onset of trouble. The longer you wait to fight back, the more paralyzed you become with fear. **When you wait, you effectively come under the spell of your assailant.**

The four inch knife he initially pulls on you will look like a sword after a couple of minutes of complying with the nut-case. *You must take action in the first few seconds.* Remember the concept of predator vs. prey: the predator expects the prey to cower and comply. When the prey attacks instead, **the predator, wounded and confused, backs off.**

It's not a bad idea to have various weapons positioned throughout your home to be used in counter-attacks against an intruder. For example, rather than keep the family's baseball bat in the garage, set it instead next to the front door. If you have a spray bottle of ammonia cleanser in the kitchen cabinet, move it instead to the area near the front door in case you need to clean the eyes of some psycho trying to break in.

Many items in your home can be used as effective self-defense weapons. If you do pick up an object to use as a weapon, **make sure you use it. Don't threaten.** Your assailant may end up using it against you if you hesitate. Remember, "He who hesitates, meditates in the horizontal position."

If there is an intruder in your home and you gain control of him, put him down. **Make sure he can not get up.** Don't think that you'll hold him under control until the police get there. At least knock him unconscious. If he is conscious and able to move, he poses a serious threat to you and your family. Remember, you are justified in killing him if need be. Have no compassion for the low-life. **Any compassion shown will be seen as weakness by the intruder, and used to your demise.** Be only concerned for you and your family.

LOCKS: I strongly recommend that you install a solid-core door both for the front and back of your property. Another good option is a metal door. A powerful home invader can easily break through a non solid-core door. However, even a two inch thick solid-core door will do you no good, if you have a cheap lock holding it shut. Sacrifice a little cash and get yourself a <u>Schlage</u> dead-bolt lock for both the front and back doors. You can also get a metal insert for the door jamb that the bolt goes into. This makes it nearly impossible to break down. Please don't get a solid-core door with *any kind* of decorative glass built into it. This type of door may look nice, but it is extremely easy to break into.

If you have a chain-lock hooked to your door, **you must get rid of it.** Even a one-hundred pound man could easily break this down, just by throwing his weight against the door. This type of lock is one of the easiest to defeat.

Sliding-glass doors, as well as sliding windows, should be secured by special locks made specifically for them. They are usually two to three dollars each and very easy to install. Without them a home invader can easily break in.

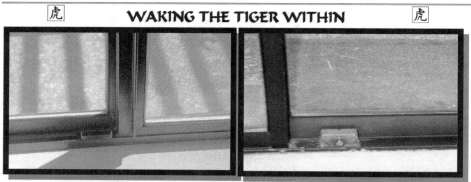

SECURE SLIDING WINDOWS/DOORS WITH WINDOW LOCKS.

CAT & DOG DOORS: Realize that if you have a cat or dog door built into one of your home's entry doors **an intruder is only seconds away from being able to get in.** He simply reaches through and unlocks the door. One way around this problem is to install a keyed dead-bolt lock that can only be turned by a key. It can't be unlocked by turning a knob. The problem with this type of lock is that if there is a fire and you need to get out quickly, without a key you may get burned.

LADDERS: **Keep outdoor ladders locked up.** A home invader can use an unlocked ladder to gain access to an unlocked window or to your roof, where he can enter through a skylight, or even an attic vent.

GARAGE DOORS: I have read scores of reports of home invasions, and kidnaps where the dirt-bag entered the home through an open garage door. Many people have fallen into the bad habit of leaving their garage door open for extended periods of time. Sometimes to cool the house down, sometimes because they are close by gardening and feel they can hear if someone approaches, or because they just forgot it was open. Please don't **make this same mistake.** Always go through the trouble of closing the garage door when you're not right there. No matter how hot a day it is or how inconvenient it may be to keep closing it, for your safety please keep all doors closed.

Dirt-bags know that home owners leave their windows open in hot weather, and purposefully **pick hot days to commit their evil deeds.** There is a cheap type of window lock you can install which allows you to lock your window in a partially open position. A home invader can get his hand through the opening but can not fit his body through.

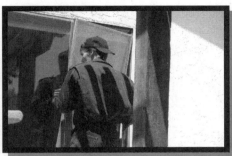 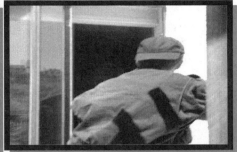

EVEN ON HOT DAYS-- ONLY PARTIALLY OPEN WINDOWS OR YOU MAY END UP WITH AN UNWELCOME GUEST.

SCREEN DOORS: If you have them, please get rid of them. **They offer you zero protection.** They are nice to have on a hot summer day, but don't think for a second that they provide any deterrent to a home invader. The only exception to this is a special security screen door made of reinforced steel. These allow plenty of air flow without the danger of an intruder kicking it down.

ANSWERING THE PHONE: If you use an answering machine, have your outgoing message say something like this: "You have reached 555-4321; we are unable to answer your call at this moment. Please leave your name and number, and we will contact you as soon as possible." Never say on you message: "We're not home right now." or, "We're away in Alaska on vacation." etc. That's an open invitation for a dirt-bag to pay you a visit.

If you have kids who are home alone either don't let them answer the phone, or tell them to let the caller know that you are unavailable at the time. **Tell your children that they must never say you are out of the house.** Instead, they should tell the caller that you are busy feeding the attack dogs, or you are rearranging your gun collection! But they must never commit that you are not home.

RESTRAINING ORDERS: At some point in your life you may feel it necessary to obtain a legal restraining order against some obsessive person who is negatively affecting your life. This is a legal instrument that bars that person from coming a pre-set distance from you. It is very important that you realize what type of effect this will have on the obsessive person your restraining order is against. **A very dangerous effect.** An obsessive person who is stalking you has it in his or her head that you are the main focus of their life. Everything in their world revolves around you.

The restraining order effectively removes you from their life. Which most often leaves them very angry, and without a purpose to live. Too often this results in the obsessive person attempting to get revenge by **trying to kill you, often followed by their own suicide.** This is commonly called "murder-suicide."

I hope you never have occasion to need to place a restraining order against someone. If you do, you must constantly be in color-code yellow, and you must follow all the principles this book teaches. **The threat of violence against you goes from arbitrary to extreme.** You don't say, "It might happen to me." You say, **" It will happen to me, most likely today, I know what to do, and I 'm going to do it."** There have been far too many people killed after obtaining restraining orders. I know first hand of a terrible death followed by suicide as the result of a restraining order.

The threat is very real, be prepared for it. Rather than the restraining order causing the obsessive person to back off, it will escalate their obsessive behavior to a new and more dangerous level. **They won't just attempt to follow you, they will attempt to kill you.** If you have to use a restraining order, put yourself on the highest stage of alert. Don't dismiss anything that seems odd or out of place. Err on the side of caution. *Extreme caution.*

Many people feel that because they live in a "good" neighborhood, they don't need to be as concerned with the possibility of attack. **Wrong answer!** *Violence can come to you at any place, and at any time.* Some nice neighborhoods are even more likely to be over-run with goblins than bad neighborhoods.

Think about it. If you were a burglar looking for a house to break into, where are you going to go, the ghetto? Of course not, you're going to go where the money is. You are going to head for the hills. The confidence which home owners in affluent neighborhoods place in not being attacked is false confidence. Especially when it comes to home invasion robberies, which are committed almost 100% of the time in the "nice" neighborhoods.

Regardless of your neighborhood **take the precautions this chapter teaches, and make your house the one that never gets picked!**

Quotes from the Group Attack Chapter

"Your mind-set during a group attack is critical to your survival. You must not let fear take over. For a short time **you must become the hunter and not the hunted."**
PAGE 68

"**Your advantage when attacked by a group is over-confidence on their part.** They are all thinking: "There's five of us and only one of him-- this is going to be easy." They also don't think that you are going to fight back."
PAGE 68

"**An armed attacker gives himself away.** When he approaches, you already know what he is going to use to try to hurt you. With an unarmed attacker, you have no idea of how he will try to hurt you."
PAGE 69

"It's a natural tendency to move back away from an oncoming attack, but that's the most dangerous thing you can do. When a goblin swings a stick or a blade at you the most powerful part of his attack is the tip of the weapon. It's moving the fastest and has the most destructive power. As you move closer to the body of the attacker his arm, in close, is moving much slower. And, if you are close in you will only be hit by the soft part of his arm and not by the weapon."
PAGE 70

CHAPTER SIX

GROUP ATTACK

Most people, when they think of being attacked, visualize a large, mean-looking person coming at them. While most often it is the case that the attacker is large, the problem is that nowadays you are more likely to be attacked by a small group than by a single assailant. Recent crime studies bear this out.

More often than not, a few of the villains will be armed. When I teach these sobering facts to my students, they are at first dismayed and alarmed. But then I teach them that being attacked by an armed group actually has some advantages over being attacked by a single unarmed attacker. It has <u>many</u> disadvantages and should be avoided like the plague, but it is very possible to defeat such an attack if you can take advantage of the inherent weaknesses of an armed group attack.

The great warrior Miyamoto Musashi often taught that once you learn to defeat a single attacker you can defeat 1000 attackers using the same technique. I believe in his fighting strategy. As long as you are fast and brutal in your technique, and escape as soon as your able, **you will survive.** The following are the principles that will keep you alive if you are attacked by a group:

BE AWARE: If you live by the color-code taught in the "Awareness" chapter, you will never be surrounded by a group of attackers. If it ever happens to you, quickly make yourself aware of the best angle of escape and move in that direction at full speed. The best way out would be to run toward your car, a store, or a street that's busy with traffic. If an assailant gets in your way, use your most lethal technique to take him out. **You can't afford for him to get back up later in the fight.** He must be totally taken out. Your best bet would be to destroy his vision or crush his windpipe. **Use full power and get out of there fast.**

Don't think you're going to be Bruce Lee and fight them one by one. In a real group attack, the goblins don't wait their turn to attack, they all hit you at once. Just like when a quarterback catches the ball in a football game, all the linebackers go after him at once. If someone else blocks your way, put him down and, once again get out of there.

Your mind-set during a group attack is critical to your survival. You must not let fear take over. For a short time **you must become the hunter and not the hunted.** You should be happy that you have four or five (victims) to attack. **Turn the tables on the vermin and surprise them with an instant, powerful attack.** By striking first, you will cause great confusion. Use this time to make your escape. And again, if someone blocks your escape route, put him down. Remember, eyes and throat.

Your advantage when attacked by a group is **over-confidence on their part.** They are all thinking: "There's five of us and only one of him-- this is going to be easy." They also don't think that you are going to fight back. Consider this-- What type of person joins a gang? A weak, unconfident person. Someone who needs to be around others to feel strong. Competent fighters don't hang out in gangs.

When you "attack the attack" by hitting first and viciously take out one of the goblins-- the remaining punks will be in shock and most likely will back down. Don't wait to see if they *do* back down. Again, **get out of there as fast as you can.**

Another tactic that can prove effective when fighting a group is to not let them surround you. When you have attackers all around you, it becomes impossible to watch them all at one time. To correct this, you simply pick the attacker who is blocking your escape route and attack him. After blinding him, use him as a screen by throwing him between you and the other attackers and then (again) run.

Many attackers nowadays carry weapons to intimidate their victims. Rather than be intimidated, I want you to be happy that your attacker is armed. Here's why: An armed attacker is a <u>weak</u> attacker. A strong fighter doesn't need to carry a weapon. While an armed attacker **puts all his confidence and attention on his weapon.** When you take away his weapon, this type of attacker will back down.

An armed attacker gives himself away. When he approaches, you already know what he is going to use to try to hurt you. With an unarmed attacker, you have no idea of how he will try to hurt you. Will he punch you with his right, or his left? Is he going to kick you? You don't know. But with the armed attacker you know he is going to try to get you with the weapon.

Here are the tactics to use against an armed attacker: First, **don't let the creep get his weapon out from where he's hiding it.** As he goes to grab the knife from his pocket, jam him up by stepping in. Use your weak hand to trap his hand going for the weapon. At the same time, use your strong hand to either attack his eyes or his windpipe. Don't play games with this type of attack. He has shown you the intent and the ability to kill you-- **put him down fast and hard.**

If the attacker has already presented the weapon and he is ten feet or more from you, your tactic is simple. **Run fast in the opposite direction.** If he has presented a gun, run and get behind cover as fast as possible. Cover would be any object that covers you from his view. When you run, don't run in a straight line. Swerve side to side to make it more difficult for him to get a clean shot.

Remember, you have many things going for you when an attacker points a gun at you. Most likely it's not loaded. Most attackers who carry guns only do so to scare their victims. Typically the gun is unloaded and the attacker has very little proficiency with it. Many times the gun is a toy or B.B. Gun.

I have taught hundreds of people how to shoot handguns under stress, and I can tell you an untrained dirt-bag will have very little chance of hitting you. If you don't take action then you might be shot, because once the creep has taken what he wants you will be close enough for him to easily get a clean shot.

If you are confronted by an armed assailant at a leg's distance, your best bet is to kick the wrist of the hand holding the weapon with a sweeping kick that travels from side to side. After deflecting the weapon, you then step toward the assailant and hold his weapon arm with your weak hand as you drive your strong hand to his eyes or his throat.

At arm's distance, your tactic is to step forward just to the outside of your attacker, as your weak hand grabs the wrist of the weapon hand and your strong hand attacks the face.

If your reactions are slow and your awareness low, you may become aware of your armed attacker while he is taking a swing at you with the weapon. Your technique will always be the same. **Always move in, never move back.**

It's a natural tendency to move back away from an oncoming attack, but that's the most dangerous thing you can do. When a goblin swings a stick or a blade at you **the most powerful part of his attack is the tip of the weapon.** It's moving the fastest and has the most destructive power. As you move closer to the body of the attacker his arm, in close, is moving much slower. And, if you are close in you will only be hit by the soft part of his arm and not by the weapon. So, always jamb an armed attacker who's swinging at you, once you're inside, again use your weak hand to grab the wrist of his striking arm while using your strong hand to go for his eyes or throat.

If the attacker has already presented the weapon and he is ten feet or more from you, your tactic is simple. **Run fast in the opposite direction.**

I hope you are never the proposed victim of a mass attack or an armed assailant, worse yet an armed mass attack. If it ever happens, **remember your advantages and be happy that your assailant is an unconfident, distracted fool as you attack his attack.**

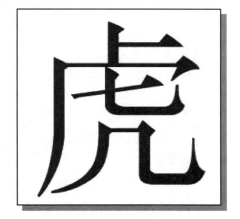

Quotes from the Travel Safe Chapter

"Always walk with energy. If your energy is low or you are sick, you must fake that you have energy. Nothing is more inviting to a goblin than a victim who shows signs of low power, or signs of being distracted." **PAGE 74**

"You must have your head up, your eyes up, and your spirits up. **A predator doesn't want to deal with someone who is feeling good.** A person like that might have the energy to pound his head in." **PAGE 74**

"Communicate to the goblin imminent death in your response. Have it be crystal clear through your body language, the look on your face, and by the tone of your voice that if he continues his evil action toward you, it will be the last action he ever takes." **PAGE 76**

"If you feel for some unexplained reason that someone is behind you, turn and be ready for a fight. It may be nothing, or you may have saved your life by not being caught off guard. **Trust your instincts."** **PAGE 78**

"Always lock all doors as soon as you get into your car. No exceptions. Just like at home, never open your door to a stranger." **PAGE 82**

"Always keep at least a quarter tank of gas. Running lower can force you to go to a gas station in an area that is too risky, or worse you can totally run out of gas and find yourself stranded in a very dangerous area. Plan when and where you get your gas." **PAGE 86**

"After parking, and **before getting out of your car, take five seconds to** look around the area surrounding your car. Never just get out of your car without checking what's happening around you. Use your mirrors, look behind you. Look for anything that seems out of place." **PAGE 87**

CHAPTER SEVEN

TRAVEL SAFE

When you step out of your home your chance of being attacked suddenly goes up, and **when you travel to an unfamiliar place that chance skyrockets.** I have heard too many stories of students and people I know being attacked when they traveled to a new, unfamiliar area. So, what are our choices then? Stay locked up in our nice, safe and secure homes? Of course not. Life is far more enjoyable when we can go where we want, when we want.

Remember, don't let anyone ever use fear to extort away your right to a happy, secure life. The whole idea of this work **is to teach you not to be afraid,** to make you aware of possible threats and to enable you to deal with them. The following are safety problems that you may experience while traveling, and how to effectively resolve them.

WALKING: When you walk, you are most exposed to the threat of violence. You don't have the protective shell of a house or car to shield you. **While walking, you must be the most prepared.** There are three principles that are crucial to your safety as you walk:

虎   虎

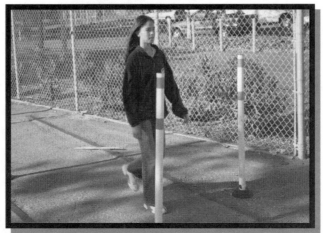

1. WALK FAST WITH PURPOSE 2. ALWAYS HAVE YOUR HEAD UP   3. CHECK BEHIND YOU OCCASIONALLY.

First, ***always walk with energy.*** If your energy is low or you are sick, you must fake that you have energy. Nothing is more inviting to a goblin than a victim who shows signs of low power, or of being distracted.

Show your energy as you walk by stepping at a good clip. Don't plod along. **Walk with purpose, as if you are going somewhere important.** Stand tall as you walk. Posture is a major body language indicator to the people around you. If you slump forward, with your eyes down and your back bent you are showing signs of fatigue, illness, depression, confusion and/or weakness, all of which dirt-bags of the world love to see in a victim.

You must have your head up, your eyes up, and your spirits up. **A predator doesn't want to deal with someone who is feeling good.** A person like that might have the energy to pound his head in.

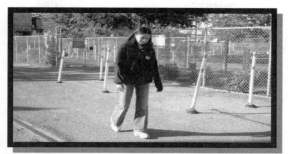

NEVER WALK WITH YOUR HEAD DOWN
IT ATTRACTS ATTACKERS LIKE A MAGNET.

Often attackers will test your energy level and the presence of fear, before they attack. Just like the dog that barks before it bites, they will be looking to see how you react to intimidation.

The most common test they will use is simply to ask a question. Often in an intimidating tone. They'll say something like, "Hey, what's the time?" or, "You got a light?" or, "You got some money for me?"

How you respond will determine whether or not you'll end up fighting the creep. Regardless of how intimidating the jerk may be, **do not let fear enter your thoughts.** Don't focus on the scowl of his face, or the fact that he outweighs you by 50 pounds, or that he is armed with a weapon. Only allow your mind to see the open targets that you are about to strike. **Be like a machine scanning for possible function targets to destroy.** Remember, no one has the right to hurt you, and the mere thought of some jerk attempting to do so should make you very angry. Show only anger in your eyes, and in your answer.

Hopefully you picked up on the possible threat of the punk while you were in yellow, and would have by now shifted to orange, ready at any moment to shift to red if the threat warrants it.

If you are really ready to fight, the attacker will most likely pick up on it and back off. If he persists with his test, answer him sharp and powerfully, while making eye contact. **Your answer is simple.** Focus extreme anger at him and say, **"NO!!",** then walk away.   Be ready to go into the fight mode if he makes even the slightest violent move toward you. When the punk says, "Man--you don't have to be so mean,"or some other equally stupid comment, just keep walking. **You owe him no explanation for your actions.** Stay in orange until the threat is gone.

With these simple techniques I'm sure you will foil the goblin's test. Even the slightest inkling of fear represents a **"Green light"** for the attacker to continue his evil plan. Stop him in his tracks with energy. Respond instantly and confidently, with **"NO!!"**

Mr. Lee would often call the actions described in the preceding chapters as **"Command Presence."** It is the ability of a person to control the actions of another through confident, forceful, loud commands. *It's not what you say, but how you say it that conveys the feeling.*

There was a study done with Highway Patrol officers of various heights and sizes to determine which characteristics are most important to control a person resisting arrest. What was found was that the power of the officer's commands had a more profound effect on the arrestee than did the officer's height and size.

The officer whose commands were obeyed most often by the test subjects was one of the smaller of the Highway Patrolmen. He was obeyed more, not because of his size but because of his conviction and the power of his voice. **There was no indecision or timidity present in his commands.** Follow this model when you respond to the test of an attacker. **Communicate to the goblin imminent death in your response.** Have it be crystal clear through your body language, the look on your face, and by the tone of your voice that if he continues his evil action toward you, it will be the last action he ever takes.

If you have some low-life whistle or yell at you from a distance, "Hey man, hold up!" or, "Hey, come here!" Just keep walking, no need to even look when called. Do shift to orange, and be ready to go to red if he gets too close. Most often the lazy low-life will give up on you after seeing that you're not going to play his little game.

The second thing to do when walking is to activate your "radar." Use your eyes well as you walk. Scan from side to side. Be aware of what's happening anywhere from one foot to one block in front of you. Look on both sides of the street. Occasionally turn your head and look behind you. Not in a fearful way, but in an aware manner. Be observant of shadows on the ground around you.

As you walk down the street look at any and all glass reflections to see who's behind you. Use the reflections like the rear-view mirror of your car. You can use store-front windows, car windows or windows on a house. The best to use are store-front windows because they are often set at a 45 degree angle, which gives a great view of what's behind you.

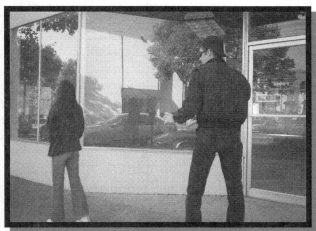

USE WINDOW REFLECTIONS TO CHECK WHAT'S BEHIND YOU.

The most common angle of attack is from behind. It makes sense because we don't have eyes in the back of our heads. But, we do have something almost as good. Many people claim they can somehow sense when someone is behind them. They say they can feel the hairs on the back of their neck standing on end, and that they get a change in body temperature, mainly on their back. This is true, it's real, and you should trust it. Your body can sense when someone is behind you.

This "sixth sense" organ is located beneath the hemispheres of the brain, and is known as the pineal gland. When this gland is surgically removed, study subjects can no longer feel when someone is behind them. Unless yours has been removed, you have a pineal gland. Trust its signals. **Don't reason them away.** If you feel for some unexplained reason that someone is behind you, turn and be ready for a fight. It may be nothing, or you may have saved your life by not being caught off guard. **Trust your instincts.**

The third thing to keep in mind as you walk is to **have your weapons ready for action.** Regardless of how cold it is, don't hinder your primary weapons of defense by putting your hands in your pockets or folding your arms in front of you. Have your hands at your sides ready to go into action.

One common mistake people make that can be very dangerous is walking with their arms full of stuff. For example, carrying two or three grocery bags at once. Goblins love this because not only are their victims weighted down by the groceries, but also their weapons of defense are out of commission. **Always have at least one hand free.** If that means making a few trips from the store to your car, or it means asking the clerk to help you carry the goods, then do it. Your planning may save your life.

Women who carry a purse should consider wearing the purse with the strap going across their body to the opposite shoulder. Doing so will make them less of an inviting target to a purse snatcher.

The following are simple steps to take while walking to help ensure your safety. Use them every time you are out walking.

When you pause, **have something secure behind you** like a cement wall, so you can be assured that no one can attack from behind.

Whenever possible, **walk toward traffic.** Not away from it. It is far better to see a trouble-maker coming toward you than be surprised by him from behind.

Always round corners wide, with at least three feet between you and the corner. Cutting the corner too tight can put you face to face with trouble, and little time to react.

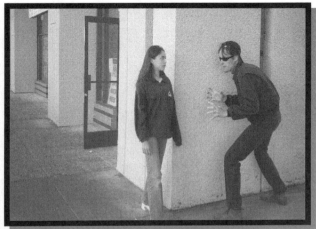

DON'T CUT CORNERS TOO TIGHTLY,
YOU NEVER KNOW WHO IS WAITING BEHIND THE WALL.

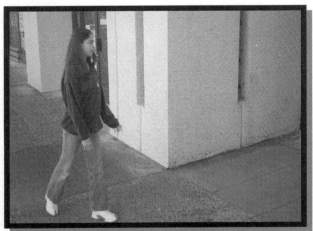

ALWAYS TAKE CORNERS AS WIDE AS POSSIBLE.

Walk down the center of the sidewalk. Being too close to buildings on one side exposes you to possible attack from a doorway. Being too close to the cars parked on the other side puts you in danger of being pulled into a car or van. Going down the center of the sidewalk gives you the most time to react to attack from either side.

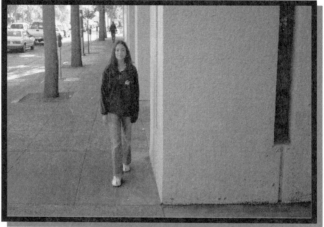

DON'T WALK TOO CLOSE TO A WALL.

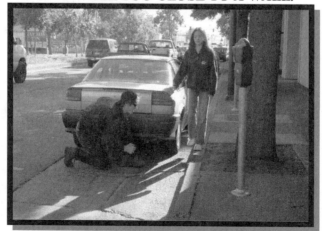

KEEP A DISTANCE FROM PARKED CARS.

Avoid using automated teller machines located outdoors. A psycho looking to rob and/or hurt someone couldn't ask for a more perfect place to attack. The person using the A.T.M. has committed three potentially fatal errors while doing their automated banking. First, odds are that while using the machine he or she is not thinking about defense. The A.T.M. user will be very distracted by the transaction at hand. Second, their back is to the street, which for most people leaves them very unaware. Third, there is money to be had, potentially lots of money. This is all too inviting to the criminal element.

The goblin concerned with being caught on the ATMs security camera can easily avoid detection by simply threatening his victim from outside the range of the camera.

Any activity that will make you unaware while walking must be avoided. **Never use headphones,** like the type used on a Sony Walkman. You won't be able to hear an attacker from behind. **Never read as you walk.** Wait till you are at a secure place before reading your favorite book or newspaper. With a book or newspaper in your face, you won't be able to see a possible threat in time. Put your priorities first as you walk, namely your own personal safety. Remember goblins attack when you are distracted.

WEAPONS: Being armed certainly gives you an advantage during a fight. There are many laws that prevent you from carrying most weapons in a concealed manner. There are a few exceptions that you should take advantage of if possible. One weapon that gives you the advantage of distance and striking force is the walking stick. It is for the most part legal to carry, as long as you are not brandishing it. If you walk with it at your side as you would with a cane, it's legal to possess. The walking stick is simply a three foot stick with a one inch diameter. **Most attackers would think twice before making a move on a person carrying a stick.**

Another effective and legal weapon is pepper spray. Mace is also very effective but illegal to carry unless you first obtain a permit. (which are not difficult to get). Both pepper spray and Mace have an instant debilitating effect on an assailant.

When sprayed at the face they cause severe pain, swelling of the mucus membranes, burning and running of the eyes, and breathing difficulties. They are inexpensive and easy to carry. You can also buy pepper spray that is more easily concealed because it looks like a writing pen or a pager.

It's a good idea to buy two. One for practice and one for actual self-defense. **You should practice spraying at a target about once a month.** To purchase these chemical weapons, try some of the self-defense product sites on the internet. Type in: **self-defense products** on your search engine.

DRIVING

As our roads become more and more crowded, three very dangerous things happen.

First, as the total number of drivers increase, so does the number of <u>violent</u> drivers who may attempt to hurt you.

Second, the more drivers there are on the road, the more congested traffic becomes, and the more frustration and anger other drivers experience.

Third, with more cars crowding the roads, there is less room to maneuver away from potential trouble.

Overall violence on the road is up 51% over the last five years.

So, how can you get around safely? It's not too difficult, you just need to learn to live by the following safe-driving principles:

Always lock all doors as soon as you get into your car. No exceptions. Just like at home, never open your door to a stranger. _Keep your windows rolled up._ If you need air, roll them down no more than two inches, or better yet, use your air conditioner if you have one. An unlocked door or open window defeats the purpose of using your car as armor against attack.

Car-jackers and rapists are experts in tricking people into opening their car door, or rolling down a window. One very common trick is the "bump and rob ploy." First the goblin bumps into you with his car, hoping you will get out to survey the damage. Once outside of your car, he's got you where he wants you.

If you are ever "bumped," here's what you need to do to survive: **Keep the engine running and the car in gear.** Do not engage the parking brake. Only use your foot brake. *You need to be able to take off instantly.* Keep a pen and paper in your glove box, so you can write down the license plate number as well as a description of the car and driver. If he wants to exchange information, cover your address and press your driver's license to the window so he can get your number. Have him do the same.

Do not under any circumstances roll down your window or open your door. There is no reason to do so. During this entire process, stay aware. Check your mirrors, watch the car that hit you to see if any passengers from the car are moving toward you. **Have an escape route planned out.** If the car that hit you is in your way, maneuver to give yourself a way out before exchanging information.

If the driver who hit you produces a weapon, such as a gun, a knife, or any object that could be used to break your car window, *immediately punch the accelerator and get out of there.* Take the time **now** to think how you will react to an armed attacker moving toward your car. Think about it so you will be ready.

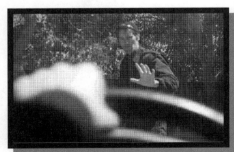 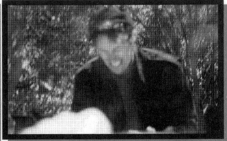

IF A CAR-JACKER WITH A GUN TRIES TO STOP YOU, KEEP GOING, DON'T STOP

Any time you drive, it is vital that you continually keep an area of space around your car for maneuvering. **Whenever you come to a stop, you must be able to still** *see the back tires of the vehicle in front of you.* This will allow you enough room to steer around the car in front. If you follow too close, you may end up trapped between the car in front and the car behind.

Many car-jackers and other vermin use this technique as a way of trapping their victims. They work as a team using two cars. The one in front slams on his brakes suddenly, then his partner in crime blocks the victim in from behind. **Don't let yourself fall into this trap.** Always keep a good distance between you and the car in front. When you stop, automatically look in your rear-view mirror to see what's coming behind you. If you see a car barrelling down on you from behind, steer around the car in front, even if that means you drive up on the sidewalk or the wrong side of the road. You must get out of that situation quickly.

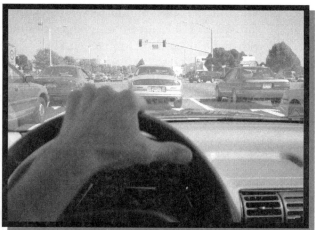

AT A STOP--YOU MUST BE ABLE TO SEE THE BACK TIRES OF THE CAR IN FRONT OF YOU.

If your car stalls, don't get out. Stay locked in your car until help arrives. This is another good reason to keep a cell phone in your car. You won't have to go hunting for a pay phone. If someone stops to help you, ask that person if he or she can call a tow truck for you. Don't open your door or window until the tow-truck or police arrive.

There is one major exception to this safety concept. If you stall on a street or freeway that doesn't have a shoulder and you are stuck in a traffic lane, **immediately get out of your car, walk toward the traffic and signal oncoming cars to avoid hitting your car.** Many people are killed each year from oncoming traffic while waiting in their cars for help.

If you get a flat tire on the freeway, **don't stop**. Reduce your speed and drive on the flat tire off the freeway. You might ruin your rim but you will avoid the danger of being hit by a fast moving car on the freeway. The best way to avoid the danger of a stalled car is prevention. Always keep at least a quarter tank of gas, keep your car tuned and in good working order, and make sure you've got plenty of tread on your tires and you'll probably never experience a stalled car.

It's wise when driving on city streets to **stay in the left lane as much as possible.** This allows you a way out if you end up in a trapped position between a car in front and a car in back. To escape this, you will have to drive on the wrong side of the street toward oncoming traffic, but at least you have a way out. If you are forced into driving on the wrong side of the street, honk your horn continually, and get back to the right side of the road as soon as possible.

Often times when in the right-hand lane, there isn't an area of sidewalk you can fit your car onto if you have to get out of a trapped situation. There are too many telephone poles, light poles, and parking meters in the way. If you are in the center lane of a 3-lane road, you can easily get trapped when traffic comes to a halt. You'll end up with cars blocking you in from all sides. Remember, on city streets your best way out is to stay in the left lane as much as possible.

While driving on the freeway, **stay in the right lane or the lane closest to the right as often as you can.** From the right lane you can access the shoulder of the road as a means of not getting sandwiched between a car in front and a car in back. Also from the right-hand lane you can easily exit at an off ramp.

At night the left lane is the most dangerous to be in. Many times drunks end up entering the freeway on the off-ramp going the wrong way. They then go to what they think is the far right hand lane or slow lane to avoid getting caught by the Highway Patrol, but they end up in the fast lane going the wrong way, often causing terrible head-on collisions. So your best bet for safe driving on the freeway is to stay to the right.

Regardless of whether you are driving on the street or the freeway, **never stop to pick up a hitchhiker, and never stop for someone who appears to be in trouble.** I know this sounds cruel and callous, but too many good people have ended their lives by stopping to help. Picking up a hitchhiker at one time was relatively safe, and stopping to be the good Samaritan was commonplace and without much danger. Unfortunately those times are long past, and to do so today could be extremely dangerous.

If you see someone who needs help, phone 911 on your cell-phone and report the problem. Or use a pay phone away from the scene. Give a good description of the person in trouble and their whereabouts, but don't stop to help. Too often it's a set up. You can't afford to chance it.

Always keep at least a quarter tank of gas. Running lower can force you to go to a gas station in an area that is too risky, or worse you can totally run out of gas and find yourself stranded in a very dangerous area. Plan when and where you get your gas. Dirt-bags often wait at gas stations looking for their next victim. A person pumping gas represents the perfect victim to most goblins. That person definitely has money, definitely has a car, and usually is very distracted, thinking of pumping gas, adding oil, or buying a candy bar. Typically the person at the gas pump is not thinking about their own safety.

A student of mine related to me a story which illustrates how dangerous a gas station can be. One bright and sunny afternoon as she worked as cashier inside the food-mart of a popular gas station, she observed a young adult male acting suspiciously near the rear door of a patron's car.

The young man was looking around in a nervous manner, as if checking to see if anyone was watching him. He then climbed into the back seat of the car he was standing next to. My student being an aware, decisive martial artist took action. First, she called 911 and reported to the Highway Patrol what she had seen. Next, she got the attention of the woman whose car the goblin had snuck into and delayed the woman from leaving the food-mart by engaging her in conversation. Within four minutes, the Highway Patrol arrived.

After interrogating the young goblin who was hiding in the back seat of her car, it was determined that as part of a gang initiation he was to kidnap a young woman, and bring her to where the gang was hiding. There, the plan was to rape her, and then he was to kill her, disposing of her body at a nearby construction site.

The goblin was found with an eight-inch hunting knife on his person, presumably to be used as the weapon of intimidation and then murder. Because this punk plea-bargained and indicted fellow gang members, he served only a short sentence and is probably at this moment committing some other heinous act.

Because of the awareness and quick action of my student, nobody got hurt. Had she not noticed the jerk sneaking into the back seat of that lady's car, that woman would have met with a horrible death. The moral of the story is: **Never leave your car unlocked, even for only a few minutes. Always check in and around your car before entering, and know that gas-stations are a favorite hunting ground for psychos.**

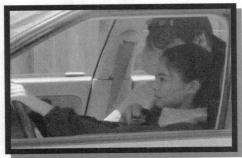

KNIFE TO YOUR THROAT...

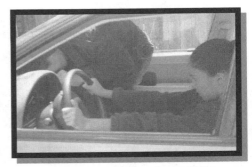

SLAM ON THE BRAKES.

After parking, and **before getting out of your car, take five seconds to** look around the area surrounding your car. Never just get out of your car without checking what's happening around you. Use your mirrors, look behind you. Look for anything that seems out of place. Look to see if someone is watching you. Many drivers have been car-jacked by attackers that were right outside their cars. Had they spent a few seconds to look around before unlocking the door, they would have seen the problem and avoided it.

Make it a habit to always spend those extra <u>**five**</u> <u>**seconds**</u> to make sure that everything is safe before getting out from the protection of your locked car. If you notice possible danger, or you get a gut feeling that something is wrong, take off and park somewhere else.

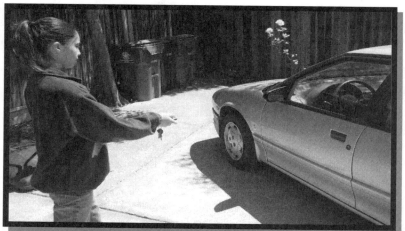

HAVE YOUR KEY OUT AS YOU APPROACH YOUR CAR.

Another good habit to instill is to **always have your keys in hand as you approach your car.** This allows you to quickly enter your car in a panic situation, and affords you a practical weapon to be used against an attacker's eyes. If you have a remote control on your key chain for your car's alarm system, you can set off your alarm if trouble is coming your way.

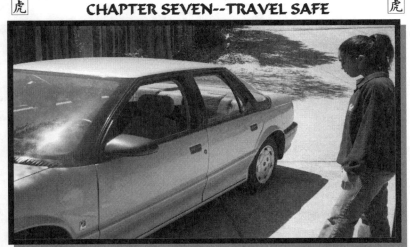

LOOK IN AND AROUND YOUR CAR BEFORE OPENING DOOR.

Always spend a few seconds **checking in and around your car before getting in.** I have heard many stories of car-jackers and rapists who wait for their victims by either hiding in the back seat of the car, or hiding outside the car opposite the approach of the driver.

When you valet park your car, **always remove your house key from your key ring.** It's also not a bad idea to take your car's registration papers with you. If you were to leave your house key with the valet, an unscrupulous person could make a copy of your house key by making a quick clay impression. That, along with your home address printed on your car's registration would give them access to your house. Sometimes the key and address are sold on the black market to the highest bidder, who then comes to pay you an unexpected visit.

Mall parking lots have a bad reputation for being popular sites for goblins to attempt car-jackings and other assorted crimes. Make it a point to always **park in a well-lighted area as close to the store's entrance as possible.** Don't hesitate to ask a mall security guard to escort you to your car if you feel unsafe walking back by yourself.

If you're ever car-jacked, you can most likely survive unscathed as long as you follow these principles:

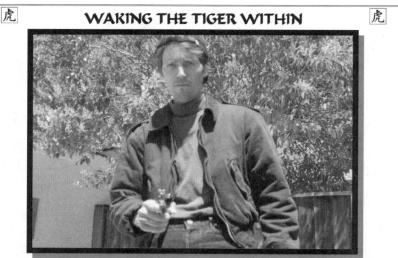

NO MATTER HOW FRIGHTENING THE GOBLIN IS-- DON'T COOPERATE.

Don't cooperate. You will be tempted by fear to go along with the program. If you sheepishly do what the attacker wants, you put him in control and will most likely suffer by his hands once he gets his way. Your best bet if confronted by an armed car-jacker outside your car is to floor the accelerator, **steer away from the jerk, and keep your head down.**

Again, I remind you I've taught many students over the years in combat pistol training to shoot under heavy stress, and what I can tell you is that most people, (even well-trained marksmen) have a very difficult time hitting a moving target. Remember, most fiends who use firearms for their crimes generally don't have them loaded, and often don't even know how to operate the gun.

If he intended to shoot you, he would have already done it. The gun is simply there for intimidation. Remember though, if you do go along with the program, after he's done with you he'll take you to a remote area and kill you there to eliminate you as a witness.

If you end up with a car-jacker in your car while you're driving, most likely the dirt-bag will not be buckled up. Make sure you are, and at an opportune time **slam on your brakes or steer into a parked car.** The sudden unexpected deceleration will throw the car-jacker through your front window. If you are being car-jacked and the goblin ends up driving, use the same technique. Make sure you are buckled up then at the right time grab the steering wheel with both hands and **steer into a parked car.** The resulting crash should give you a short time of confusion in which to make your escape.

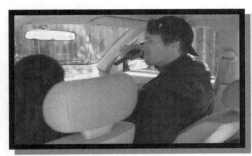 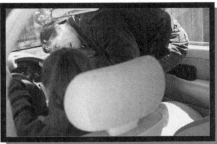

CAR-JACKER TAKES CONTROL,   SLAM ON THE BRAKES--STOP THE GOBLIN.

If you become overpowered by a car-jacker who locks you in your own trunk, **you must get the attention of the police.** Most likely the goblin has locked you in the trunk to drive to an area where he can dispose of you without any witnesses. **You must get help before it's too late.** There will be very little light, if any, in the trunk. Feel around for any wires or cables. Rip with all your might at any wires you find. Don't stop with one. **Rip out every wire you can find.** Hopefully you'll rip out a wire that powers the car's fuel pump, brake light, turn signal light, license-plate light, etc.

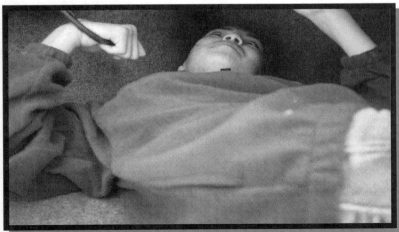

ONCE INSIDE THE TRUNK RIP AT EVERY WIRE YOU CAN FIND.

You may be able to find the cable that releases the trunk. If you think you have it, wait for the car to stop and then pull with all you've got.

If none of the above has worked, get ready for a fight. Get your feet positioned near the locking end of the trunk, rest your back just below your feet, so you are essentially upside down. As soon at the goblin unlocks the trunk to get you, **explosively kick with both legs on the trunk lid, shoot your legs out of the car as you press with your hands to spring to your feet.** Most likely the trunk lid will have hit the goblin, or at least surprised him enough to buy you two or three seconds of confusion, in which you **attack his eyes.**

Remember, he doesn't expect you to fight back, so when you do he will be very confused. The reason he will be getting you out of the car's trunk will certainly be a terrible reason. Don't wait to find out what it is. **Take charge and fight for your life.**

ROAD RAGE

A relatively new term that refers to the angry, stressed-out way some people get when they are behind the wheel of a car. You could have your life severely shortened if you react incorrectly to a driver experiencing road rage.

When you are confronted by a driver under the influence of road rage, the number one thing you'll probably say to yourself is: "Man-- is that jerk over-reacting." All you did is beep your horn to have him speed up, and next thing you know he wants to kill you!

The over-reaction is the result of one (or both) of two things. First, regardless of the driver's physical size or level of fighting skill, **he feels invincible with two tons of steel wrapped around him,** and because of that sense of security he takes on a "Dr. Jekyl/Mr. Hyde persona." Once inside his car no one better do anything to make him angry.

The second ingredient that sets road rage into motion is one small incident that caps off a mountain of built-up stress. The stress is often from having to drive in overcrowded rush-hour traffic, getting cut off by other drivers, or from rushing to get somewhere with too little time.

When you give the friendly little beep of your horn to get the guy to go, it becomes **"The straw that breaks the camel's back."** And, in an instant Dr. Jekyl becomes the hideous Mr. Hyde, ready to drive you off the road or ready to pull out a gun and blow your head off.

The following are methods to employ as you drive so that you can avoid being the catalyst that puts another driver over the edge and into "Road rage."

PARKING: Many people each year are killed fighting for parking spaces. Most of these fights are for a parking space close to the store. Rather than walk another twenty feet from an open parking space, they instead fight to the death for the closest space. If you find yourself in a similar circumstance, just let the maniac have the space and walk the extra twenty feet. The exercise is good for you.

DON'T BE IN A RUSH: When you are hurrying to get somewhere, you will invariably anger other drivers. You'll end up tail-gating, cutting people off, changing lanes without looking and without signaling. All of these are avoidable simply by giving yourself more time to get where your going.

NO TURTLES ALLOWED: If you are driving ten miles per hour under the posted speed limit, you are going to really anger the majority of drivers, who are typically in a rush. Driving too slow is one of the major causes of road rage.

BE THE WILLOW, NOT THE OAK: Don't offer resistance to threats and angry gestures. Temporarily swallow your pride. I know this runs exactly opposite to everything taught earlier in the book, but *you are in a completely different world when on the road.* In a face-to-face confrontation **strength equals peace.** If you are confident and strong in your resistance, your attacker will most often back down.

But, in a road rage situation the tables are turned. The crazy driver experiencing road rage has a powerful suit of armor protecting him **and will not be intimidated by your show of force.** You should give him the right-of-way, get out of his way, and avoid him like the plague. Don't give him any excuse to attack. If he gives you the extended middle finger, or shakes his fist at you-- let it go. It is definitely not worth it to get involved. Just pretend that you didn't see it, and put as much distance between you and him as possible.

If things get really bad and he is already committed to hurting you-- then **you must take defensive action.** Whatever you do, don't stop and get out of your car to confront the creep. **Keep your suit of armor around you by staying in your car.** Drive away from the nut as fast as you can while still keeping your car under control.

Drive to the nearest police or fire station. If you have a cell phone, call 911 and alert them to your situation, and give them ongoing updates on your location. Once you get to the police or fire station, honk your horn repeatedly to get their attention. **Don't stop, and don't get out of your car.** Keep driving by until you get help.

Gun shots are fired at your car by a maniac with road rage-- what should you do? Keep your head low and keep driving. If he is following you, at an opportune time, **slam on your brakes,** causing your assailant to crash the front of his car, then speed off as fast as you can. Remember, most people are not very accurate shots, especially when trying to shoot a moving target. As long as you keep moving, your chances of being shot are extremely low. **If you stop to fight, you will most likely be shot.** Keep driving until either he gives up or you get help.

HOTELS/MOTELS

Unless you're lucky enough to stay at a friends or relatives home when you travel, you'll probably end up in a hotel, or worse yet a motel. The problem with hotels and motels is their appalling lack of security. The same dangers you read about in home safety dealing with your home, exist when you stay at a hotel or motel, only they are far worse. The following ideas will help you to have a safe and secure time while staying at a hotel or motel.

Don't tell anyone you are alone: Even if it means you pay more for the room, don't tell the staff that you are all alone. Many unscrupulous bell boys and clerks have used the knowledge of a customer staying alone to commit the crimes of rape, burglary, and even murder on their unsuspecting guests. Let the staff know that your family or friends will arrive at any time soon.

Insist on a secure room: You will not accept a room on the ground floor. You won't accept a room that has a door to an adjoining room. There must be a lock on your door that once you're inside cannot be opened from the outside. There must be a peep-hole on your door allowing you to see who is at your door. Of course don't open your door to someone you don't know, even if that person claims they are part of the hotel's staff. Try to have a floor plan of the hotel sent to you when you book the room. This will give you a chance to plan the best escape route from your room if there is trouble.

Give your room "the once over" before going to bed. Confirm that there are no unwelcome guests staying with you.

Even with the above security items taken care of, you must go one step further by **alarming your room.** The best way to do this is to buy a cheap $10.00 motion detector to place on your door. If anyone even bumps into your door while you are asleep, a loud ear-piercing siren will go off waking you up and giving you a little time to prepare to fight. You can arm this type of device as you are leaving your room. Then, if someone tries to enter your room while you are away, the entire hotel will know about it. Realize that the cleaning staff will come into your room each day to clean, unless you put out the "do not disturb" sign.

RESTAURANTS/PUBLIC PLACES

When ever you walk into a public building like a restaurant, movie theater, courthouse, bank, etc., always think: **Where is the nearest exit?** If there was a sudden attack by a nut with a gun, you would know exactly how to quickly get away from the danger.

When sitting at a restaurant, **always sit with your back to the wall at such an angle that you will be able to see the entrance door.** Try to sit near an exit. If you can't be near an exit, consider breaking a window with one of the chairs to make your own exit in the event of an attack on the restaurant.

With your back to the wall, you will not be attacked from behind. With a clear view of the entrance door, you will be able to see an attacker before he strikes. These tactics for sitting at a restaurant are age-old in the martial arts, and are done to protect the highest-ranking person or source of information.

ELEVATORS

Modern day life almost guarantees that sooner or later you will find yourself riding on an elevator. There are some goblins that use elevators as their place of attack. Just being aware of this fact may save your life. If you ever get the gut feeling that the guy looking at you from inside the elevator is trouble, **don't under any circumstances get in.** Just turn and walk away. You can always wait for the next one. If you happen to find yourself alone in an elevator with someone who gives you the creeps, do the following:

Press the next floor's button so you can get out quickly.

Position yourself near the doors, with your body in front of the control panel with at least a peripheral view of the goblin. If the jerk wants to press the emergency stop button in order to attempt an attack, he will first have to get past you. If you are panicked, press as many of the different floor buttons as you can so, you'll have many chances to get out.

Stand tall and be ready to spring into action. Visualize in your mind a vicious attack to the goblin's eyes and throat.

Don't dismiss your gut instinct that something is wrong about the person in the elevator with you. Don't rationalize your danger radar away. Your subconscious has most likely picked up some signals that your conscious mind has not yet registered. All you have is an uneasy feeling, but you can't put your finger on what or why. Once again, don't question it. **Trust it and get out of that elevator.**

TOURISTS

The most dangerous time in your life, when you are most likely to be attacked is when you are traveling in an unfamiliar area. **Tourists are the favorite prey of the goblins of the world** for the following reasons:

They are easy to spot. Tourists make the mistake of not blending in, wearing clothes that stand out. Shorts in a climate where everyone else is wearing pants. Brand-new clothes with bright colors. A camera around the neck, and a generally lost look on the face.

They're not armed. It is illegal to carry most weapons on common carriers such as airliners. Goblins know this and purposefully go after the tourist.

Tourists make the mistake of flaunting wealth. They wear expensive jewelry, and carry large amounts of cash.

False sense of confidence. When people travel from developed countries such as Japan, the United States or England to third world countries they incorrectly assume the country they are visiting has the same overall safety as the developed country. Those tourists are often unpleasantly surprised at how dangerous the country is that they are visiting.

Tourists are assumed to be rich. People in most third world countries don't have the money to travel. So they think that anyone who can travel must be rich. They often resent that supposed wealth, and are willing to take drastic action to take it from tourists.

So, what's the answer? Never travel to new areas? No, that would be an awful way to live your life. Travel is fun and exciting, and no matter what the possible threats are, you shouldn't let a few dirt-bags ruin your fun. The key is to **avoid trouble by not standing out as a lost, vulnerable tourist.**

Learn about the area you will be traveling to. The more familiar you are with the new area, the more confident you will be as you stroll down the street. Use the Internet to get maps of the area, and information on the sights you want to visit. Find out as much as you can about the culture of the people you will be visiting. Your primary goal is to blend in.

Find out what people usually wear in the area you will be visiting. Hopefully you will already have similar clothes. It's best not to wear brand new clothes.

Go with a group if possible. There is strength in numbers for tourists. Being with a group is especially important if it is your first time to the new country. A tour group is a great way to go because the tour guide will only take you to areas that are "safe" for tourists. Don't venture out on your own, unless you know for certain the area you are going to visit is relatively safe. Stay in the neighborhoods that are set up for tourists.

Consider arming yourself with weapons that can be carried on common carriers. A good solid three foot walking stick is an example. A goblin would think twice before trying anything with you carrying such a weapon.

Don't carry cash. Use credit cards, or travelers checks. If they are stolen, you can get them replaced. If you normally carry your wallet in your back pocket, change it to your front pocket. Pickpockets have a very hard time getting your wallet from the front. Carry a little extra cash in your sock or shoe, just in case you need some emergency money.

Don't tempt fate. Even if you think you are in a very safe area, don't leave valuables out in plain sight. Some desperate people might attempt to kill you in order to get your valuables.

Whenever you travel you must **continually be in color code yellow.** If you slip into white, you could find yourself in serious danger.

By using the aforementioned concepts you should be able to have a safe, enjoyable trip with little chance of being attacked.

Quotes from the Growing Up Prepared Chapter

"No one can protect your child from the monsters that kidnap and molest children, **except you.** The judicial system routinely releases the goblins who commit these crimes to go out and ruin more lives. The police can't be everywhere at all times. But, **your fighting spirit can.** Imagine how hard you would fight to save your child from a kidnapper. Then teach your son or daughter to **fight as hard as you would fight for them.**"
PAGE 104

"**Talk to your child about defense from kidnappers as often as you talk to your son or daughter about his or her grades.**"
PAGE 104

"No matter how smart you think your child is, **an adult kidnapper is going to be smarter and able to trick your child,** if your child makes the mistake of talking to a stranger. The rule is simple-- **DO NOT EVER TALK TO A STRANGER.** "
PAGE 105

"**Kidnappers don't want a fight.** That's why they pick little kids as their victims. When the child fights back, the kidnapper in most cases gives up, and quickly makes a get away. There have been many accounts where **just minimal resistance has caused the abductor to give up his evil plan. It is crucial that the child fights the abductor immediately when threatened.**"
PAGE 112

"**5 MINUTES TO SURVIVE:** Everything goes wrong and the kidnapper gets your child in his car. **He or she must escape within 5 minutes.**"
PAGE 113

"As you're shopping, keep things in perspective. What is more important in your life, your child or looking at the ingredients on a spaghetti sauce can? **You must look out for your child at all times.**
PAGE 116

CHAPTER EIGHT

GROWING UP PREPARED

3 00,000 children in the United States are abducted each year, **46,000 never to be found again.** This is a tragedy that can be prevented. Other children are terrorized everyday at school by bullies, often causing permanent psychological damage which effects the rest of their lives. Why are we as parents, friends and family allowing this to happen to our kids? Is it laziness, apathy, or ignorance on our part?

It's actually none of the above. Instead, <u>denial</u> is what puts our nation's kids at risk. Just like with our own personal safety we want to believe that it only happens to other people, but never to us. We want to think that our children are somehow exempt. To think otherwise is too awful a thought. So, we pretend that the danger doesn't really exist.

The danger is real, and we must prepare our children for it. This chapter will teach you effective techniques of prevention and defense for dealing with abductors and bullies. Your kids then need you to teach them, and they need you to continually go over this information with them.

I strongly recommended that you as a concerned adult go back and re-read the preceding chapters. They deal with keeping *you* safe. The safer you are, the safer your children will be when they're with you. This chapter will teach you basic principles to keep your children safe when they <u>can't</u> <u>be</u> <u>with</u> <u>you.</u>

Remember the danger is real! In terms of percentages, the chance that your son or daughter will ever be abducted is low. But, percentages are cold comfort if your child happens to be the one in 1,000 that is abducted. To really keep your child safe, you must go into this with the presumption that **your child will be attacked and that it will happen sooner than later.** I know it's a terrible thought, but this is necessary to be really prepared. To do otherwise will weaken your approach to teaching these crucial self-defense concepts.

What kind of monster abducts a child and why? The vermin that go around hunting children are angry, disturbed individuals who want to hurt someone, but are too weak and cowardly to pick a person their own size. **They are often sexual deviants who rape their victims prior to killing them.**

Not long ago there was a classic case of abduction ending in tragedy that illustrates how evil and twisted these criminals are. In a small Arizona town, a petite ten-year-old girl was walking on her way home from school. Her parents allowed her to walk to and from home alone because they lived in a **"nice neighborhood"** where everyone knew each other. She felt tired as she walked the eight long blocks from school to home. So, when the nice man offered her a ride, she readily accepted. He won her confidence as he had with all his victims by **smiling, dressing well and by talking with a soft, kind voice.**

Once inside the car, she came to know the real monster he was. He immediately grabbed her arm. She went for the door release, but it didn't work. She screamed for help, **but it was too late.** No one could hear her with all the windows rolled up. He then punched her in the temple knocking her unconscious. At least now she wouldn't feel the horrible pain inflicted on her as he repeatedly raped her over the next four hours. She only came to in time to experience the worst possible terror of being thrown off a bridge 100 feet to her death.

A jogger found her naked at the bottom of the bridge curled in the fetal position, gravel clenched in her fists. She had survived the terror of the fall only to die an agonizingly slow death from her internal injuries, cold and alone in a washed-out gully.

We know these facts because the perpetrator was later caught trying the same evil scheme on another ten-year-old girl. Only this time, **she had been taught what to expect, and what to do.** When he offered her the ride, **she ran,** later giving police a detailed description. He had a long criminal record with many sexual crimes and prior kidnappings. He was out on parole when he raped and killed the little Arizona girl. He confessed to everything, giving a detailed description of his heinous act.

Let us not allow her death to be in vain. If this story has made you angry-- **I know it made me very angry--** take that anger and use it for good, by teaching the children you care for to have **an indignant attitude against these goblins.**

Midsy Sanchez's mom did and eight-year old Midsy is alive today thanks to her mom's constant reminders of how to deal with abductors. Midsy's abductor overpowered her as she walked home from school in her Vallejo, California neighborhood. She normally walked to and from school with her brother, but on this particular day, he wasn't there to walk her home. She decided to walk by herself.

Nearby, the 39-year-old goblin was waiting. He had been paroled only nine months earlier after having served a reduced sentence for kidnap. Once he got Midsy in the car, he overpowered her. He then drove her 40 miles south to San Jose. The kidnapper had Midsy shackled by the ankle. Over the next two days, he continually terrorized and raped her.

On the second day of her ordeal, the goblin briefly left Midsy alone shackled to the car. As soon as he was some distance away, Midsy scrambled to find the key to unlock the shackle. Once free, she ran as fast as she could. The kidnapper saw her and gave chase. Midsy kept yelling: **"He kidnapped me-- I'm Midsy Sanchez-- He kidnapped me!"** She was able to flag down a truck driver before the molester could catch her. Shortly after Midsy gave her story to the police, the goblin was found and arrested.

The goblin that kidnapped Midsy had been in jail eleven times before, and he had a long rap-sheet. Many people believe he may also have been responsible for the disappearance of another eight-year-old Vallejo girl, who was taken on her way to school.

Brave Midsy is alive today because her **mom constantly went over with her how to defend against an abduction.** Had Midsy not ran when she did, the kidnapper would most certainly have killed her.

It was a chore for Midsy's mom to keep reminding her of the dangers of kidnappers and how to escape their attacks. **But, that effort was well worth it. And, now children everywhere have a hero to copy.** Just three weeks after Midsy's ordeal, a little girl was grabbed at a Target store in Cupertino.

Her response to the 40-year-old goblin who grabbed her was to **slap his face and scream at him, until he let go and ran like the coward he is.** Many children and parents have learned from Midsy's plight, and they are making the whole business of child abduction difficult--**good for them.** If enough children fight against these monsters, I think we will find a return to the relative safety of the 1950's and 60's for our children.

We are always reviewing safety issues with our children; we remind them: "Look both ways before crossing the street," and "Don't play with matches." However, the one most important safety point that **does not get pushed enough** is how to be safe from the threat of abduction. It's an awkward subject and it takes energy to constantly review with your child the danger associated with strangers. But what is the price paid for being silent? It may be a very high price-- not knowing were your child is, not knowing if your child is alive or dead. **That's torture to any parent.** If you don't teach and remind your son or daughter how to stop an abductor, then you may pay this awful price. *Please talk to your child about kidnappers.*

No one can protect your child from the monsters that kidnap and molest children, **except you.** The judicial system routinely releases the goblins who commit these crimes to go out and ruin more lives. The police can't be everywhere at all times. But, **your fighting spirit can.** Imagine how hard you would fight to save your child from a kidnapper. Then teach your son or daughter to **fight as hard as you would fight for them.**

The following concepts must be constantly reviewed with your child. We are creatures of habit and we only remember those things that we hear over and over again. Self-defense principles need to be part of your child's character. This can only be accomplished through lots of repetition. **Talk to your child about defense from kidnappers as often as you talk to your son or daughter about his or her grades.**

Remember the more prepared your child is to defend against a kidnapper the less likely he or she will ever be picked as a victim.

Don't feel that you are stealing your child's innocence or childhood by going over the realities of kidnapping with him or her-- If you don't, **your child's innocence and childhood might permanently be taken away by some goblin.**

The basic idea of this chapter is not to scare your child; instead the idea is to empower him or her with knowledge. To inform your child of the possible dangers, without teaching how to fight against those dangers, would be cruel. The child would be left frightened of threats with no method for fighting back. Your child must be taught the dangers, but in the same lesson-- **how to overcome those dangers.**

Here are the ideas you must get across to your child. Test the retention as you teach by always following up your instruction with questions. Play the "what if game" with your child often. Ask: "What would you do, if----?" Praise the right answers and gently correct the wrong answers.

It's good to be rude: Teach your child to be rude to strangers. Not polite. **Polite kids get kidnapped.** Rude kids don't. It's easy to be rude. All your child has to do to be rude to strangers is **not to talk to someone he or she doesn't know.**

No matter how smart you think your child is, **an adult kidnapper is going to be smarter and able to trick your child,** if your child makes the mistake of talking to a stranger. The rule is simple-- **DO NOT EVER TALK TO A STRANGER.** I know this sounds mean and callous, but it is necessary. The only exception to this rule is if your child is already under attack by an abductor. Then and only then should your child talk to a stranger and only in order to get help. Midsy Sanchez did, and the stranger she flagged down helped to save her life by driving her away from the goblin.

Kidnappers rarely just come up to a child and grab them; instead they first try to engage the child in conversation. This starts the insidious process of taking control of your child. **The process must not be allowed to start.** As long as your child knows never to talk to a stranger under any circumstance, **he or she has just reduced the chance of being kidnapped by 90%.** Only around 10% of the time does a kidnapper just grab a child without first trying to talk the child into going with him. If the parents of that little Arizona girl had taught her to be rude and to never talk to strangers, she would most likely be alive today.

The following are just a few of the lines kidnappers use to trick children:

"Can I give you a ride?"

"Can you tell me where Main Street is?"

"I lost my little kitten, can you help me find her?"

"Your name is Tina-- right?"

"Remember me?-- I'm a friend of your father."

"Your mom asked me to pick you up. She's hurt-- I need to drive you to the hospital to see her."

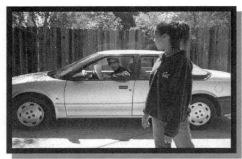
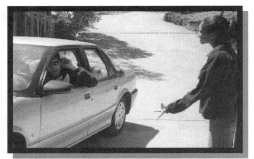

"CAN YOU TELL ME WHERE MAIN STREET IS?   *COME CLOSER, I CAN'T HEAR YOU..."*

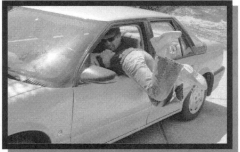

AFTER BEING TRICKED INTO GETTING TOO CLOSE,
THE VICTIM IS GRABBED BY THE GOBLIN.

Every word the child utters in response will be used against him or her by the kidnapper. **If your child says nothing, he or she shuts down the plan of the goblin, and most often the kidnapper gives up** and searches for a more gullible child.

A few years ago, the Oprah T.V. show did a very good segment on how to teach children to stop abductors. They showed how easily a young child can be tricked by a stranger. The segment was filmed at a park full of children having fun playing. The camera man set up his shot so that the viewer was able to see Oprah interviewing the mother of a child who was playing behind her in the background.

Oprah asked the mother: "Do you think your son would ever talk to a stranger, and if he did, do you think he could be tricked by a kidnapper?"

The mom emphatically said NO. She said her son had been taught to never talk to a stranger, and that if he ever did, he knew better than to ever <u>go</u> with a stranger.

While this was being filmed, in the background the viewer could see a stranger talking to her son, and after only about ten seconds her son went with the stranger.

Oprah asked: "Where is your son right now?" The mother turned her head to look behind her and said: "Why he's right there...." To her amazement he was gone.

Luckily the man who had tricked her son was a undercover police officer there to show how easily a child can be tricked if he or she talks to a stranger. The officer and her son were only around the corner and the boy was quickly returned to his very shocked and relieved mother.

So, what's the answer? The boy in the above example was taught to never talk to strangers, but he did and was tricked into going with the stranger in just ten seconds. Obviously, the mom thought she had done a thorough job teaching her son. What she had neglected to do **was to continually remind her son of the anti-abduction concepts. Remember, you need to** *go over these ideas with your child as often as you talk about school.*

Random kidnappings by total strangers are very rare. More often the kidnapper knows something about the victim. They often know the child's name, where he or she lives, the school the child attends, or the name of the child's parents. All this information is used as ammunition to win the confidence of the child. But it won't work on your child, because **your son or daughter will not speak to a stranger, no matter what.**

If your child tends to be an extrovert and is very sociable and talkative, you need to enforce the no-talking to strangers rule even stronger. The advantage of the extroverted child is that they are usually not afraid of strangers. This lack of fear helps to repel kidnappers. The problem with the extrovert child is since they like talking to a stranger, he or she is open to being conned by a kidnapper.

I want my daughter and son to grow up to be polite, well-mannered adults. They are taught to be very polite and respectful to our family, but they know being rude by not talking to strangers is what we expect of them. **This is the main protective concept you can give your child.** If they know it and use it, they have taken away the principal weapon of the kidnapper.

WHAT DOES A STRANGER/KIDNAPPER LOOK LIKE? I often ask my young students this on their first lesson. The common responses are: "A kidnapper wears a mask," or "A kidnapper has a mean face-- with a beard and mustache." And " Kidnappers wear black clothes." The reality is quite the opposite. Once again, over 90% of abductions start with the kidnapper first talking to the child. The last thing the abductor wants to do is to scare away the victim. So, they do whatever they can to look nice, speak softly and dress normally. They want to win your child's confidence, so they purposefully look as "normal" as possible.

How does your child know who is and who isn't a kidnapper? It's simple. **Anyone he or she doesn't know must be considered a potential kidnapper.**

Your child must understand that even the friendly neighbor you wave to each morning while taking your child to school is a stranger-- and must be thought of as a kidnapper. Many parents will read this instruction and think,

I don't want my child to have to go around thinking that each and every stranger is a kidnapper. They don't have to teach this concept to their kids. They can try a more "even-handed approach" where their child is left to sort out who is and who isn't a kidnapper on his or her own.

But, the bottom line remains that simplicity is key. If your child has to make value judgments based upon some complex system of what strangers probably are and what strangers probably aren't kidnappers, the resulting confusion may cause him or her to guess wrong and end up falling into the trap of an abductor. **You've got to keep your instruction simple and clear or your child won't use it.** If your child knows that all strangers must be thought of as kidnappers, he or she won't take the unnecessary risk of trusting a stranger, and wont end up in trouble. **Keep it simple.**

Of all the safety rules that you teach your child, **not talking to strangers is the most important.** If your child forgets everything else taught in this chapter, but remembers: **DO NOT EVER TALK TO STRANGERS,** this one concept by itself will keep your child alive.

STRANGE FEELINGS: Teach your child to trust his or her "gut instinct." If your child gets a "strange feeling" about someone, no matter who it is, teach him or her to **trust that feeling,** and get as far away from that person as possible. Children have a stronger survival instinct than we adults do. Kids have not had a lifetime of denying their "gut feelings", so they are more aware when danger is present. Tell your child to embrace this gift of instinct, and to **never ignore it.**

Even people your child knows can turn out to be bad people. There have been countless rapes, molestations and kidnaps committed by people the young victims knew as a relative, neighbor, teacher, counselor, doctor, priest, dentist. **This is where instinct can save your child's life.**

If your son or daughter gets a strange feeling about someone they are with, **regardless of who it is,** they need to trust that feeling and act on it. He or she should get away from that person fast, and your child should tell you about it right away.

I have heard of too many cases where a child has survived a brutal ordeal and then reported that he or she had sensed a bad feeling about the goblin who hurt them right from the beginning. **If only people would trust their "gut feelings," we would have far less victims.**

REPORT TROUBLE: You need to teach your child to let you know instantly when something strange happens to him or her. If you notice that your child is acting withdrawn or depressed, it may be the result of an encounter with a child molester who hurt him or her.

Goblins who release their young victims after molesting them often tell the victim that if they say anything about the incident, they will come back and kill the child, or they will return and hurt or kill the child's parents. The victim is so intimidated by this that they don't report what happened and often are continually molested for years after. Or, the child carries the emotional scars of the attack for a lifetime.

Let you child know that this technique of intimidation is just one of the molester's tricks and that **nothing will happen to him or her or to you when your child tells you.**

Teach your child to let you know if someone touches him or her on the areas covered by a bathing suit, or if an adult or big kid takes their clothes off in front of your child, or if someone threatens your child in any way.

How prevalent is sexual molestation of children? **One out of three woman report that they have been sexually molested at some time in their life.** Most say it happened when they were little. It's probably close to that same rate with young boys. Remember, your child should tell you immediately when something strange happens to him or her, or if your child gets a strange feeling about someone he or she needs to first get far away from that person, and then to tell you about it.

THE LINE OF ACTION: Teach your child not to allow a stranger to get closer than six feet from him or her. If a stranger gets that close, your child will be in extreme danger. At a distance of five feet or less, a stranger could easily lunge forward and grab your child.

Six feet sets the line of action. If the stranger crosses that line, your child should back away re-establishing the six-foot safety zone, all the while watching the goblin. If the attacker charges, your child will have enough room to maneuver and run away.

Practice with your son or daughter where six feet is. Rehearse the action of your child moving away as you move closer than the six-foot line. If you charge forward, your child should practice running and screaming: **"Kidnapper-- that's not my dad-- Kidnapper!!!"** Saying "that's not my dad" is important because a person seeing a youngster being grabbed by an adult may assume that the adult is the parent just trying to control a temper tantrum. Teach your child: **Run, scream, get help.** Run inside a store, go to where there are lots of people. Don't stop running until you are safe.

FIGHT FOR YOUR LIFE: No matter how frightened your child is when attacked, he or she must fight. If a stranger ever tries to grab your child, **the instantaneous reaction must be to fight, and to fight hard.** Teach your child to break from a wrist grab by quickly making a big circle with his or her arm, to get loose, and then to run. Practice this wrist grab technique with your child until it works every time. Teach that if the goblin bends over to grab your child, **he or she should instantly strike the attacker's eyes.** Review "the stop button" chapter with your child. Get him or her a styrofoam wig head to practice eye strikes on. Remember, teach your child to **strike, run, scream, and get help.**

If your child is grabbed in such a way that he or she can't get to the eyes, the next tactic is to bite the grabbing hand hard and run. Carefully practice this with your child. Tell him or her not to really bite you. Teach your child how to kick the groin and the shin. Hold out your hand as a target. Your child should eventually be able to kick your hand nine times out of ten. Teach your son or daughter how to use the elbow and knee as a striking weapon for when the attacker is close.

Play the grabbing game with your child. See if you can grab and carry your child all the way across the living room before he or she can break free. If you can get all the way across the living room with your child, then so could a kidnapper grab and drag your child into a car. Practice until your child can **escape your grip before you can travel the distance of your living room.** You may get a little beat up during these lessons, but you will be **teaching your child a skill that may someday save their life.**

Kidnappers don't want a fight. That's why they pick little kids as their victims. When the child fights back, the kidnapper in most cases gives up, and quickly makes a get away. There have been many accounts where **just minimal resistance has caused the abductor to give up his evil plan. It is crucial that the child fights the abductor immediately when threatened.**

The longer the child waits the less likely he or she will ever be seen alive again. This is because the more time that passes once the abduction has begun, the more frightened the child becomes. The fear causes a type of paralysis. The child in effect falls under the spell of the kidnapper. Also, the longer the child waits to fight, the further the kidnapper will drive away from the child's familiar surroundings.

THE LAST RIDE: Your son or daughter must understand that if an abductor pulls him or her in his car **it will be the last ride your child ever takes.** The purpose of the car in an abductor's mind is control. Once he has the child in his car, he has that child under complete control. Nine times out of ten he will take his victim to a remote location to rape and then murder the child. Your son or daughter must know this and **must be prepared to fight for his or her life to avoid the goblin's car.**

Your child must equate the abductor's car with death. **Don't sugar coat this concept, give it to your child straight.** If this point is under-emphasized it won't be used, and you may lose your child. Please don't gamble with this one.

While being pulled into a car by a kidnapper, your child may as well fight with everything he or she has. Fighting right at the start allows for the chance of someone coming to help, and if your child loses the struggle at least the end will come without the torture of having first been raped. If he or she waits until the goblin has reached a remote location to fight--it will be too late. There won't be anyone to help, and your child will be more afraid than ever because the kidnapper would have had a long period of time to terrorize your child on the way to the remote location.

You've got to push this point with your son or daughter the hardest. No matter what, your child must not go in a stranger's car. **He or she must bite, scratch, scream, kick, spit, elbow, knee and cause such a ruckus that the abductor gives up and drives off. Many young lives have been saved by simply resisting. Your child won't do it unless you push it.**

5 MINUTES TO SURVIVE: Everything goes wrong and the kidnapper gets your child in his car. **He or she must escape within 5 minutes.** After 5 minutes two very bad things happen. First, 5 minutes is enough time for the kidnapper to reach the freeway from the residential area where he took your child from. Once on the freeway most hope is lost. Escape is nearly impossible at freeway speeds, and secondly the further the goblin takes your child away, the more difficult it is for searchers to find him or her.

In most cases searches are conducted nearby where the child was last seen. In the case of Midsy Sanchez, she was rescued over 40 miles away from where she was taken. It was only by her own accord that she was able to be rescued. There were no searches to speak of being conducted in the San Jose area where she was found.

How can a small child escape from an abductor's car? **Any resistance is good resistance.** Fighting gives your child a chance. The goblin is taking his victim to die, so fighting will not worsen things for the child. The best technique is to jump out of the car when the car stops at a stop sign. **Even jumping out of a moving car is better than waiting to die.**

Another effective technique is to cause the car to lose control and crash. Teach your child how from the passenger seat to grab the steering wheel and to pull down with both hands causing a severe right turn. On city streets this would most likely result in a collision with a parked car. This will at the least create some attention to the kidnappers car. At best it will disable the vehicle and thwart the plan of the goblin. Your child could be injured from the collision, but once again, at least fighting will give him or her a chance.

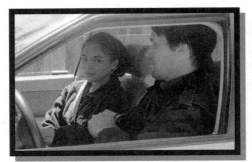

KIDNAPPER GAINS CONTROL

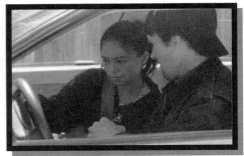

SHE PULLS WHEEL HARD TO RIGHT

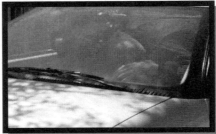

THE CAR CRASHES CAUSING THE UN-BELTED GOBLIN TO HIT THE GLASS.

Teach your son or daughter to quickly, from the passengers seat of the car, hit the throat of the goblin below his adams apple with the side of the left hand. This should be done with a fast hinging motion off the elbow. Practice this by holding out your hand and having your child chop your hand, hard. The resulting crushed windpipe will cause the abductor to loose control as he gasps for air. Remember, It only takes 4 to 5 pounds of pressure per square inch to crush the windpipe. An average **four-year-old can hit that hard.** All this must be done within the first 5 minutes, before getting on the freeway. Remember, teach: **strike, run, scream, get help.**

THE TRUNK: It's very common for abductors to try to get their young victims in the trunk of the car rather than in the passenger area. The thought is-- if the child is in the trunk no one will see that the child needs help and no one will interfere. Take some time to teach your child what to do if he or she gets locked in the trunk of an abductor's car. Now is a good time to review the chapter, "Travel safe." There you will find a section that teaches how to escape from a car's trunk. The best way to teach your child how to escape is to use the trunk of your own car. During a car-jacking your child could end up in the car's trunk and it would be a good idea for him or her to practice how to get out.

PAGE 114

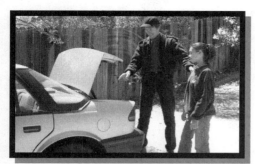

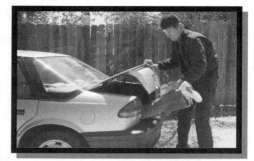

"LOOK-- A KITTEN... "   *CHILD GETS THROWN IN TRUNK.*

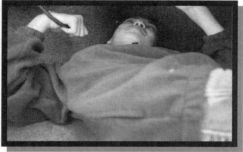

ONCE INSIDE THE TRUNK, THE CHILD SHOULD PULL ALL WIRES/CABLES.

The first thing to teach is once again, fight and create a scene before being pushed into the trunk. Once inside it will be dark and disorienting. Your child should immediately start feeling for wires or cables. He or she might get lucky and find the cable release to the trunk. The cable is usually on the trunk lid near wear the key goes in. He or she should feel for the center of the lid and then find the back of the trunk lid nearest to the rear of the car. Show your son or daughter where the cable is on your car as a reference. See if he or she can make your car's trunk lid release. Your child should wait till the car stops and then should pull that cable hard. If the trunk opens: run, scream, get help. If it doesn't open, your child should keep searching for wires.

Any wire gets pulled hard until it breaks. After breaking one, he or she should search for more to break. The idea is that if enough wires get pulled, sooner or later some of the car's rear lights will go out. Even in bright daylight a car will be pulled over if its brake lights don't work. **This technique has saved a number of lives.**

Kicking at the sides of the trunk and at the trunk's lid should be done every time the car stops. The concept is to get attention. If the abductor stops to silence the child, this represents a second chance at survival. As soon as the jerk opens the trunk lid, your child should know to instantly kick up on the lid, and to drive a finger into the eye of the kidnapper, then: **run, scream, get help.** Waiting is not an option. All of these techniques must be executed before the car hits the freeway.

SHOPPING WITH KIDS: Talk with your child before leaving your car to remind him or her what you expect of them while you are shopping. Kidnappers know that children often leave their parents while shopping and wander off to areas like the toy section, the candy section, the food court, etc. To avoid this happening to your child, you have to make an agreement with your child that you will take them to the area they want to see as soon as you are done with what you need to do. Always follow up and take them when you are done.

As you're shopping, keep things in perspective. What is more important in your life, your child or looking at the ingredients on a spaghetti sauce can? **You must look out for your child at all times.** It is a terrible feeling to look back to where you last saw your child and see that he or she has vanished. You get an awful feeling in the pit of your stomach. If this should happen, instantly search for your child. Check first the areas your child would want to go see. Next head to the front of the store to ask if your child has checked in with them. Listen carefully for your child's voice. **Don't call out your child's name** as this can be used against your child by a kidnapper. The goblin can trick your son or daughter by calling him or her by name.

Your child should know that if separated from you, he or she should yell out your name continually until you arrive. The next thing for your child to try would be to go up to the front of the store and ask one of the adults wearing a store uniform if he or she can page for you over the public address system. **Under no circumstance should your child leave the store without you.** The only stranger he or she is allowed to talk to is a person wearing the store uniform.

NAME TAGS/BACKPACKS: It's not a good idea to write your child's name on everything he or she wears. It's also not good to write the name on a back-pack or lunch pail.   Kidnappers have an edge on your child when they know his or her name. Kids tend to trust strangers who know their name. Don't make it easy for a kidnapper by writing your child's name on everything.

Backpacks have been to blame for a handful of kidnappings in the past. These children fell victim to kidnappers who were able to easily catch them because the child couldn't run fast enough to escape carrying their backpack. They were told by their parents to not lose their backpacks, no matter what. So, when the kidnapper gave chase, these poor children tried to run away with fully-loaded, heavy backpacks. Tell your child that if he or she is in danger and needs to run, the first thing to do is drop the backpack. The children who were caught by their attackers were all grabbed by their backpacks. I remember hearing the parents interviewed after the children had been molested, but found alive. Those parents felt terrible.

HALLOWEEN: This should be a fun, exciting time for your child, not a trip to the emergency room or worse, being kidnapped. Here are a couple of things to keep in mind to protect your child: **Always go with your child while he or she trick-or-treats.** Go up to the door with them, every time. Allowing your child to go trick-or-treating with an older sibling or an older friend is not safe. You are always going to be the best person to protect your child from harm.

Halloween has a bad reputation for being a time when a lot of kids get hurt. **Survey any and all treats that are put in the bag before your child eats them.** It's not a good idea to have your child eat candy out of the bag while trick-or-treating. It's too difficult to see in the dark what type of candy is about to be eaten.   Every year there are reports of children who are poisoned by tainted candy, or injured by candy or fruit that has had sharp implements such as razor blades put into them. You should always spill out the contents of the goodies bag on the floor in bright light and separate out any suspicious looking items. Don't let your child eat any raisins, peanuts, apples, or any fruit. Candy with a twist wrapper should be thrown out. Only completely sealed candy should be eaten. The safest approach is to throw out all the candy in the bag, and buy your own goodies for your child.

INVITING GOBLINS INTO YOUR HOUSE: No matter how effective a security system you have, no matter how well locked up your house is, no matter how big and bad of a dog you have, it's all worthless in keeping out kidnappers, sexual deviants, child molesters, and the like. Because the moment your child goes on line using the internet, these scoundrels of society come right into your home, maybe even into your child's bedroom. Many children every year are kidnapped or molested by goblins that they meet "on line." The main group that is being victimized are young girls, ages 11 to 16. **This can be prevented.**

Whether you have a son or a daughter, and regardless of your child's age, you must protect him or her from these monsters. Here's how: The simplest approach is to not allow your child to go on line unsupervised. You can insist that your child not go on a "chat line." Many molesters pose as children on line while "chatting" with your child. They find out your child's name, where he or she goes to school, and sometimes even where your child lives. All this information is later used against your child by the molester who, armed with the child's name, school location and home address stalks the child, waiting for an opportunity to attack. Or even worse, the molester arranges to meet your child at a public place and then commences to molest him or her.

Under no circumstance should your child ever give out personal information on line such as: his or her name, address, school, grade, age, your name--unless he or she checks with your first.

You should check the internet history window on your computer to see what web-sites your child is viewing. If your child uses e-mail, you should have full access to it. No passwords (unless you know them). If any of the above is a problem for your child, the answer is simple. Either disconnect internet service, or only have it available to you. Your help button can give you information on how to arrange a password to restrict your child's use of the internet.

There are many great sites on the web that your child can benefit from. The main dangers of the internet lie in the chat-rooms and in some web-sites. Your safest approach is to only allow your child to use the internet while you are right there.

TEACHING KIDS: In this chapter I have tried to cover all of the possible ways of protecting your child from the horrors of being abducted or molested. There is quite a lot of information to get across to your child, **all of it very important.** I suggest that you not try and get all this to your child in one lesson. Instead try to teach one concept per week. During the week, review it often. Ask questions to make sure he or she is getting it. Praise the correct answers. Play the "what if" game as much as possible. Ask, "What would you do if you were shopping with me and suddenly you couldn't find me-- what would you do first?"

It's vital when teaching children that immediately after you make the child aware of a possible threat, you also teach him or her **how to defend against the danger.** You don't want a scared child. Fear breeds attack. You want your child to be "street-wise." To know what dangers exist and to know that he or she can handle such danger.

I have taught thousands of children to defend themselves throughout my teaching career, but it is my hope that with this book, parents like yourself will spread this instruction to many more children than I could ever reach by myself. And you are always going to be the best teacher for your child. Perhaps, years from now, **if enough children start fighting back against the evils of kidnap and child molestation, the whole business of these goblins hurting kids will stop.** Growing up in such a time would allow for a happier childhood for our kids, and I certainly look forward to that time.

Quotes from the Putting An End to Bullies Chapter

"What can you do to help your child if he or she is being bullied? If you are going to choose to under-react or over-react, it's vital that you over-react. Remember, the problem must be stopped immediately."   **PAGE 122**

"School should be a pleasant learning experience for your child. If he or she is being tormented everyday by a bully there is little chance that your child will do well in school."   **PAGE 123**

"**Bullying is always an escalating venture.** It starts out usually with name-calling. Just like the shark that bumps it's prey before attacking, the bully will be checking to see if there is fear in his proposed victim. If there is, he or she will continue with more and more humiliating attacks." **PAGE 123**

"Tell your child that when it comes to bullies, **you expect him or her to fight back and that you will support your child's actions 100%.** Many kids never fight back against bullies because they are afraid they'll be in trouble with their parents, and they allow the bully to harass them for many years."   **PAGE 124**

"Instill an indignant attitude in your child toward bullies. **Instruct your child to not let an aggressor get away with anything.** Should a bully attempt to torment your child, he or she should instantly fight back, and then again go straight to the principal to report what happened and to call you. Cause a stink, get results. If your child doesn't immediately fight back, the hesitation will be interpreted as fear and will cause the bully's attacks to get worse.   **PAGE 125**

CHAPTER NINE

PUTTING AN END TO BULLIES

Bullies must be stopped early on before they can do too much damage to the physical health and self-esteem of their victims. Almost every adult has at one time in their life had a problem with a bully. Whether they solved the problem, or let it continue, had a profound effect on the rest of their life.

Those adults who as children let the bully continue to terrorize them, most likely had a difficult time at school and probably allow co-workers or family members to bully them as adults. The adults who as children fought back against their tormentors most likely continued to have that same indignant attitude toward all future bullies, and were for the most part never the victim of a bully's attack again.

All predators have the same line of thinking. If the prey shows fear, attack. **If the proposed prey fights back, find some other prey that won't.** Bullies are no exception to this. A bully can only exist if his victim allows the bullying to progress. As soon as the victim fights back, the bully suddenly backs off. This is because **bullies are at their core cowards,** with a low self-image. They feel that they have to continually dominate those around them to feel any self-worth.

Secure, confident people don't go around looking for fights. Because they are not threatened by others, they can be calm and peaceful with people around them.

Bullies can terrorize at any age. Many adults need help in fixing abusive relationships where a spouse or a co-worker physically or mentally torment them.   However, the focus of this chapter will be on helping children. Children have the most to lose from being bullied, because it can ruin their entire lives.

How do you know if your child is being bullied? What are the signs? Here are some things that should key your attention:

An - A - student rapidly drops to a - C - student.

Bruises or cuts that your child blames on other things.

A general depressed view of life.

A sudden unexplained aversion to wanting to go to school.

Vanishing lunch money.

Getting in trouble for fights that your child swears he or she didn't start.

All of these signs spell trouble, and need to be investigated further. You as the parent need to put lots of attention on solving the problem. If you ignore it, your child could at the least suffer lower self-esteem, poor grades, little self-confidence and a future of the same. At worse, your child could be physically hurt, **or could even be killed.**

What can you do to help your child if he or she is being bullied? If you are going to choose to under-react or over-react, it's vital that you over-react. Remember, **the problem must be stopped immediately.**

Talk to your child to find out who the bully is and what he or she has been doing to your child. This may be difficult, because most kids are ashamed to let their parents know what awful things have been done to them. You must press on and find out all the details. Either the same day you find out, or early the next morning go to the school and talk to the highest-ranked person there (probably the principal) and **scream bloody murder.**

Once again, over-react. If you are gentle in your approach with the school, little if anything will be done. Demand that the bully be taken out of that class, or expelled from the school. Threaten law suits against the school and against the parents of the bully if there is even the slightest bullying against your child. If you don't get results go to the school board, pursue legal action.

Make life a living hell for the bully that attacked your child. Your son or daughter will probably hate all the attention you are putting on the situation, but for sure they will thank you for it later, and it is your primary job as a parent to protect your child from harm. Follow up after your complaint to the school. Ask your child if the bullying has stopped, go back to the school over and over again until you get what you want. **No one messes with your child.**

School should be a pleasant learning experience for your child. If he or she is being tormented everyday by a bully there is little chance that your child will do well in school.

Bullying is always an escalating venture. It starts out usually with name-calling. Just like the shark that bumps it's prey before attacking, the bully will be checking to see if there is fear in his proposed victim. If there is, he or she will continue with more and more humiliating attacks, such as throwing objects like spit balls, paper airplanes, rocks and bricks. Use of liquids such as glue on the chair seat, paint on the chair seat, throwing milk. Spitting on the victim, spitting in the victim's food. Damaging the belongings of the victim. Writing on the books, breaking into the victim's locker, stealing personal items of the victim. Physical blows to the victim. Kicking the shin, the groin, the body, Punching the stomach, the face, the shoulder, the back. Shooting the victim with everything from a sling-shot to a shotgun.

I recall in fourth grade seeing a kid get his head slashed open. As he was bent over to get a drink from the water fountain, the bully kicked him in the rear driving his face into the water faucet and a brick wall. The victim had to get twenty stitches. The bully got a detention.

It can get really bad for your child if you let it. Bullying is not limited to school. It often happens in the neighborhood, at the park, at after-school programs. There will always be bullies around your child. **Don't let your child be the victim.**

BULLY PREVENTION: Stopping the problem before it becomes a problem is always the best tactic. Here's what you should teach your child to help them to deal with bullies: Make sure your child understands that no matter how big and scary looking the bully is, he or she does not have the right to hurt your child and that the bully is being a bully because he or she is insecure and is a coward. **You've got to give your child the confidence to stand up to the bully.**

Most all schools have a zero-violence policy. If a child fights, that child gets sent home. Tell your child that when it comes to bullies, **you expect him or her to fight back and that you will support your child's actions 100%.** Many kids never fight back against bullies because they are afraid they'll be in trouble with their parents, and they allow the bully to harass them for many years.

Teach your child to over-react to the threat of a bully and to follow these guidelines: If some kid calls your child a bad word, he or she should look the bully right in the eye and angrily command **"Stop It!"** Immediately after, your child should go to the principal. Yard monitors for the most part won't be of much help. Your child needs to go right to the top. If on a subsequent occasion the bully physically touches your child in any manner, your child should very forcefully slap the bullies hand off, and with eye contact and a pointed finger-- command loudly "Don't **EVER** touch me again!!"

Teach your son or daughter to have a defiant attitude toward bullies. He or she should become very angry when a bully attempts physical contact. Your child should then go straight to the principal's office to complain, and call you at work or home. Once again, this should be made a very big deal.

It has to be so painful for the school when a bully tries to hurt your child that everyone at the school goes out of their way to prevent it from happening. **If you under-react nothing will be done.** Schools are run as a bureaucracy and for anything to get done, you first have to get noticed. You and your child need to cause a major ruckus every time there is a problem with a bully.

If it happens again that the bully physically touches or harms your child, instruct your child to snap kick the bully in the groin full power, and then to stand over the bully and say "You were warned, next time I won't be so nice!!" Then again, right to the principal's office.

Your child might get suspended for the day. But, it will change two people's lives forever and will be **well worth it.** Your son or daughter will be changed because he or she will have learned to fight back, and with the confidence gained from the experience, your child will most likely **never be targeted again as a bully's victim.** Your child would also have done the bully a big favor. The bully would have learned that it's not a good idea to go up to people and pick on them. If the bully hadn't learned this lesson with your child, he might have continued to bully people for many years. As an adult, the bully might go up and harass an armed person who may not be as forgiving as your child was.

Bullying for a junior high school or high school student can be a very dangerous proposition. The bully/victim relationship is basically the same as it was in elementary school, but now the bullies are much bigger and stronger and are capable of extreme damage. Especially in junior high school the amount of bullying and fights increase dramatically. Most likely this is due to the onset of adolescence.

Young adults try to establish a "pecking order" at this age. To make sure your child doesn't end up on the low end of that order, here are a few things to help: It's better to have friends than enemies. Encourage your child to have as many friends as possible. Try to get your child to get involved in team sports, and in some of the clubs available in junior high and high school. In general, kids with a strong core group of friends don't get picked on much.

Once again, instill an indignant attitude in your child toward bullies. **Instruct your child to not let an aggressor get away with anything.** Should a bully attempt to torment your child, he or she should instantly fight back, and then again go straight to the principal to report what happened and to call you. Cause a stink, get results. If your child doesn't immediately fight back, the hesitation will be interpreted as fear and will cause the bully's attacks to get worse.

Do your child a big favor and teach them not to stand for being bullied-- **not now, not ever.** This martial artist attitude will give your child a happy, rewarding time during school and for the rest of his or her life.

Embrace the Tiger...
Abandon Fear

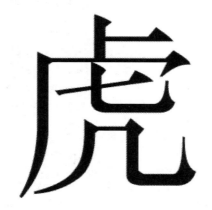

Chapter Ten

Terrorist Beware

Having read the preceding chapters on your personal security you are already prepared to deal with most all possible terrorist threats.

In the *Awareness Chapter* you learned how to use mental conditioning and the color code to be ultra-aware of your surroundings and how to trust your gut-instinct.

The *Tiger Chapter* dealt with the emotional state-of-mind needed for brutal self-defense. (definitely the most difficult and most vital self-defense trait to learn.)

Then in the *Stop Button Chapter* you were taught the secrets to ending a fight in one second as well as devestating self-defense techniques.

In the *Home Defense Chapter* your house was transformed from a simple dwelling into a sanctuary. You learned to defend your home as an extension of yourself.

The *Group Attack Chapter* helped prepare you for the ever more common gang-attack. (*Chances are if you're ever attacked it will be a small group.*)

In the *Travel Safe Chapter* you were taught all you need to know on moving about in a safe, secure way.

It is now time to discuss the ever-present and growing threat of terrorism. You are most likely to encounter terrorism as you travel. Whether your travel is walking around your own familiar neighborhood or touring in a foreign country you are exposed and more likely to be the proposed victim of terrorism.

Terrorist as the name implies rely on their targets being easily terrorized. The average un-trained individual will nine times out of ten cower with fear when unexpected violence comes their way, playing exactly into the plans of the terrorist.

Because of the training you've received by reading **Waking The Tiger Within** you won't be shocked or surprised when terrorist violence comes your way. Quite the opposite. You expect it and will most likely act against the terrorist **before** he can move against you.

Many people have asked me: "How can I protect myself from a totally random terrorist attack like a Suicide-Bomber, where the terrorist walks into a crowded area and sets off a bomb?"

The answer is, you can't avoid every possible terrorist attack. It may happen so unexpectedly that you just can't escape. In that case the terrorist gets you, but he only wins if you allow yourself to be so fearful of a potential attack that you let that fear alter your normal lifestyle. You've got to take reasonable precautions; beyond that you are falling into their trap by allowing a potential act of brutality to terrorize you.

In the case of the Suicide-Bomber, there are some possible ways to defend against even something that extreme.

Number one: As always, trust your gut-instinct. If all of a sudden you get the feeling you're in grave danger, don't wonder why. Immediately evacuate the area while you prepare yourself to take defensive action.

The gut-feeling reaction was caused by a definate danger. Your sub-conscious mind picked up on a signal that your conscious mind had not yet registered.

While at the restaurant you spotted out of the corner of your eye a very desperate, nervous looking man walking your way. It was just a glimpse, but it was enough of a danger signal to trip the adrenal system controlled by your sub-conscious into high-gear, shutting down your digestive system and resulting in a queasy feeling in the pit of your stomach. We call that your "gut-feeling."

You don't know why you feel it, but you know something is wrong. By trusting your gut instinct you'll be able to get away from the desperate, nervous man heading your way. He's desperate for a reason. He's going to blow himself up for his "Cause", hoping to kill as many Americans as possible. You won't be one of those Americans because you are long gone when he self-ignites.

Number two: It's important to be vigilant. Any time you're in a large group setting you are more of a target for terrorism. While at an arena, movie theater, restaurant or any other area where you're grouped with many other people you must be extra aware and alert. **Know where the exits are.** Try to stay at the periphery avoiding the middle of the crowd. Watch for people behaving oddly, and stay focused on those who don't seem to fit.

We are all very fixated lately on protection from terrorists while flying. After the hijackings of September 11, 2001 it makes sense to at least be weary of such attacks happening in the future.

Flying The Not-So-Friendly Skies

It is definitely more frightening to fly since the attacks of "9/11." The government has made an attempt to increase security for America's flying public, yet few people feel any safer flying even following the recent safety procedures implemented.

I feel we are actually safer flying now than at any other time in our country's history, as passengers today are all very aware of any suspicious behavior from a fellow passenger and any form of aggression is instantly squelched.

Before September 11th, most airline passengers gave very little attention to the people around them and assumed that the worst thing that could happen during a flight would be a hijacking to divert the flight to Cuba or some other third world country, and **as long as everyone cooperated, no one would get hurt.**

As we have all recently learned, ***the rules have changed.***

No longer will "going along with the program" guarantee survival. In fact just the opposite. Now passengers are prepared to take matters into their own hands, taking responsibility for their own future.

If someone onboard does anything even slightly threatening, they are instantly pounced upon and subdued by fellow passengers. ***This is the main safety characteristic that has changed since "9/11."***

Think of all those poor souls aboard the planes flown into the World Trade Center and the Pentagon who lost their lives due to everyone onboard those ill-fated flights just "going along with the program."

Lucky for all of us, that will never be allowed to happen again.

The passengers aboard the flight that crashed in Pennsylvania had it right. They knew that the hijackers were going to use their flight to kill innocent people as in the reports they had heard from family via cell-phone calls. They knew that if they did what they were told they were going to die anyway. So, they decided to fight back. Because of their brave sacrifice, they most likely saved hundreds of people at the White House from being killed. Today most everyone on any flight has that same attitude of fight for your life and never submit.

Passengers now are ready and willing to fight back against terrorists who threaten them. There is no safety procedure or device that measures up even slightly to this major safety improvement. There is today in effect a plane full of Sky-marshals ready to take action.

What Can I Do To Be Safer?

Number one: Be an aware passenger. As soon as you get onboard, take a look around and determine who might be likely to cause trouble.

Watch for things that look out of place. Like the recent incident with the Shoe-Bomber taking off his shoe and then trying to ignite some part of it. Luckily a stewardess was paying attention and instantly threw hot coffee at his face allowing time for surrounding passengers to tackle him before he could set off a shoe-bomb. It was later shown using an actual airliner that had the shoe-bomber been able to detonate his device, it would have blown the plan into two huge pieces, instantly killing all on board.

Number two: If possible arrange to sit near or at the back of the aircraft. There are several tactical advantages to being at the very back of the plane. First, the rear of the plane often survives the perils of a plane crash. You are certainly going to be near an exit, which could be very important if the plane is commandeered while still on the ground. The most important reason is to be able to see what the aggressors are doing at all times. You don't want one of those crazies at your back.

Number three: Look around you to see what improvised weapons you can find to defend yourself.

It's unlikely that a terrorist will be able to bring a firearm onboard to commit his awful deeds. Probably you will need to defend yourself against a fanatic who is wielding a small sharp implement such as the box-cutters used on "9/11."

In such an instance, you must create an improvised weapon that will give you a distance-advantage and act as a shield against an edged-weapon.

Here are some common items onboard an aircraft that can be used as defensive weapons:

- 1. Your belt (a good long-range weapon.) It's easy to quickly take off your belt and use it as a vertical blocking device held between both hands. After blocking a stabbing attack, you can wrap the belt around the attackers wrist and pull him off balance.

- 2. A cup of steaming-hot coffee or tea (thrown at the face stops most all attacks.) Remember, this was used quite effectively against the Shoe-Bomber.

- 3. The fold-down tray in front of you can be broken off and used as a shield. With the tray in the extended position, you can drive both forearms down with full force breaking it off and then use it to deflect an attack.

- 4. Your blanket, pillow, jacket or other piece of clothing can be used as a cushion wrapped on your weak arm to take the blow of the terrorist's sharp implement, leaving your strong arm free for a counter-attack.

- 5. Your shoe thrown at the attacker's head can create a momentary distraction.

- 6. A women's purse (a great long range weapon) can be swung at the attackers head, or used to deflect an attack.

- 7. Your briefcase or laptop computer can be used as a shield or blunt weapon swung at the head.

- 8. The credit-card phone in front of you can be thrown or swung at the attacker's head.

- 9. A rolled-up magazine can make a strong stabbing weapon directed at the throat.

- 10. Your seat cushion, and life preserver can easily be removed to make a great deflection device and shield you from a stabbing attack.

Its easy to see that most anything can become an effective improvised weapon when one has the correct mind-set for survival. The important thing to keep in mind is that you are fighting for your life. So, anything goes, and your counter-attack must be sudden, fierce and as unexpected as the terrorist's initial attack.

I hope that more people return to flying knowing that now, because passengers are ready to take responsibility for their own safety, the skies may not be friendlier, but they are at least much safer.

Using the principles taught in the preceding chapters you will be so aware that you will see danger before it strikes, and if a would-be-terrorist tries to make you his victim, you will be able to instantly turn the tables on him.

It's time that we as a society become so prepared for trouble that we make the terrorists beware.

Let's get the point across to the terrorists that we're mad as hell and we're not going to take it anymore.

Time To Unleash
The Tiger

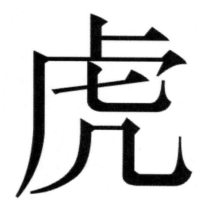

AFTERWORD
(A FEW FINAL THOUGHTS)

How likely is it that you will ever have to use any of the concepts taught in this book?   Unfortunately, **it is very likely.**   Our world is a dangerous place, full of threats ranging from an angry person cutting you off on the road, to a gang of attackers attempting to kill you. The big problem is that due to our population growing so fast, the threat of violence is getting worse. In the relatively short amount of time that I've been around, the world population has almost doubled.

With so many people crowding our limited resources, we are experiencing more and more violent crime. As the population continues to grow, there will be large increases in violence as a whole.

Take any population of animal species, double it's population within the same given space and you won't have a doubling of violence, you will have a **quadrupling in the incidents of violence.** We as humans are no different when it comes to overcrowding and violence. So the bad news is, we can expect more threats of violence as time goes on. I wish this weren't the case, but sadly it is.

The good news is that people who commit violent acts on others are always looking for an easy victim. After taking the instruction of this book to heart, **you will by no means be an easy victim.** You will have learned to be very aware, you will have learned countless ways of preventing the possibility of attack, you will know how to carry yourself, how to be safe while at home, at work, and when you travel, you will even be prepared for a terrorist attack.

You will know that your children are safer because of the prevention steps you have taught them, and because you know they will fight back effectively if attacked by a kidnapper.

Many well-intending martial arts instructors as well as some police will instruct their students that there are times that it is wise to submit, comply or follow the commands of an attacker. They will say that if you are clearly outnumbered or if your attacker is armed you should do what he says, that you should cooperate to avoid getting hurt.

I know these teachers mean well, but they are setting their students up for a possibly *lethal failure*. When most people are attacked their first reaction is fear. If they have been taught that they have a choice between fighting or not fighting, almost 100% of the time they will choose to not fight. Not because the situation warrants compliance, but because of fear. The student is left with an option of submitting due to fear. This concept causes the student to have an inherent weakness in their fighting strategy. The result is that the student has fear in their heart. This fear is picked up on by goblins and attracts them like a magnet to steel. Rather than this helping the student, the compliance concept actually makes it more likely that they will be attacked. **Please don't adopt this fearful way of thinking.**

After reading this book, I hope that you will understand that you have only one choice, and **that is to fight**. So, when fear kicks in at the onset of the attack, your only response, (the only response you know) is to fight. When you have the mindset of always defending yourself no matter what the attack, you experience a rather nice paradox. **No one wants to attack you.** The goblins of the world can see that **you are a *Tiger* and want no part of you.**

Aside from all the methods of prevention you have learned, the most important concept I hope you will have gained from this instruction **is how important it is to fight back.** If you have it firmly planted in your mind that, yes, if you are attacked, regardless of the odds you will fight back, then you will have acquired a new inner-strength, a new inner-peace, and you will have **awakened the tiger within.**

About the Author

Scott Flint, a 5th degree Black Belt, holds the title of Master Instructor, has taught over 4000 students during 31 years and has learned from experience exactly what women, men, and children must know to be safe in all environments.

Scott is also Senior Chief Instructor of West-Wind Kung-Fu Schools in California. He is Director of the Taipei Chinese Kung-Fu Association United States Of America Branch. Besides traditional Kung-Fu, Scott teaches a course in Personal Protection using the Combat Pistol.

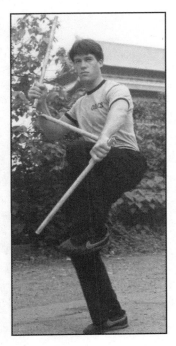 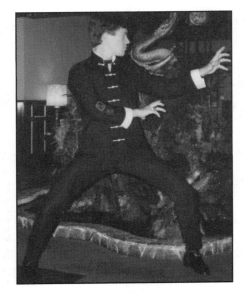

The author training in China.

With a true to life self defense book like Waking The Tiger Within, you too can Learn Effective Self Defense, gain valuable Tips, Tricks and Advice whether you are a man or women in minutes!

Caroline from Detroit Michigan writes, *"Dear Parthenon Press, Scott's concepts are fantastic. Now, without even joining a class, all women can learn to protect themselves from situations that can unexpectedly occur anytime and anywhere. His book is so clear and easy to understand. It is a must for every woman!"*

"I travel for business a lot and bought Waking The Tiger Within, thinking it would be good to have that kind of knowledge – especially these days. My whole family ended up reading it, and I even sent it to my daughter who is away attending college. We are all so glad she read it. Just last month a would-be attacker was "Easily deterred as my daughter put it. She sent the guy running – probably to the hospital! Anyway, thanks from all of us,"
The Halloways
Sonoma, CA

"Don't fight fair ... fight to win!" Do you know what two traits will almost always save you in a threatening situation? Attitude and Mental Toughness. Waking the Tiger Within shows you how to "get your mind right" so you will be in control -- and not a victim. 5th degree Black Belt Master Instructor, Scott Flint has taught over 3,000 men, women and children how to be safe in all enviroments. This is NOT some dull karate, judo or kung fu instruction book. A MUST read!
Linda Wallis, CEO--Personal Security Marketplace.com

"The way in which the book is organized is really great, flows easily and is hard to put down."
Edward A. Ipser, Jr., PhD
President and CEO, CivilShield.com

"Just finished your book. Two thumbs way up!"
In the Arts,
Tim Walker Sr

"What I like about Waking the Tiger Within is that it teaches the attitude and mental toughness necessary for defense."
Michael Gravette, President, Safetytechnology.com

What a GREAT book! For those like myself and my wife, who have long ago eclipsed Jack Benny's 39 years, and who are also handicapped, staying safe in a violent world is not easy. Martial arts? Try them with Degenerative Joint Disease. We knew there had to be a better, easier way for those of us long past our prime "fighting years".

As a volunteer personal safety instructor, I read, watch videos and attend as many seminars and programs as possible, always looking for ways to keep ourselves, and others, safe.
"Waking the Tiger Within" by Scott Flint has to be one of the best sources of staying safe to come along in some time.

The book covers not only the number one ingredient of safety, ie awareness, but guides the reader into developing "Your natural built-in instinct to survive". His chapter, "Stop Button" is exactly what we have searched for: ending "an attack in one second." (No gun, pepper spray or Black Belt needed.) Worth the price of the book by itself.

Got kids or grandchildren? Worried about bullies? His chapters on these subjects are excellent.
Road Rage? Car-Jacking? (What would YOU do, if locked in the trunk of your car by an assailant?)
Many of the areas Scott writes about are covered in the seminars I present, but this book opens up a host of new, and surprisingly simple, techniques that almost anyone, at any age, in any state of health, can grasp and use.

Chapter One begins with these words: "No one ever has the right to hurt you." When you have finished reading and following the simple advice presented in these pages, you will be a long way toward the realization of that goal. Buy this book for yourself and give copies to those you love.

P.L. Schoentube, N.R.A. Certified Instructor for the Refuse To Be A Victim Program, Sherrif Deputy Morgan County, Great Cacapon, WV

Also Available from Turtle Press:

Defensive Tactics
Security Operations
Vital Leglocks
Boxing: Advanced Tactics and Strategies
Grappler's Guide to Strangles and Chokes
Fighter's Fact Book 2
The Armlock Encyclopedia
Championship Sambo
Complete Taekwondo Poomse
Martial Arts Injury Care and Prevention
Timing for Martial Arts
Strength and Power Training
Complete Kickboxing
Ultimate Flexibility
Boxing: A 12 Week Course
The Fighter's Body: An Owner's Manual
The Science of Takedowns, Throws and Grappling for Self-defense
Fighting Science
Martial Arts Instructor's Desk Reference
Solo Training
Solo Training 2
Fighter's Fact Book
Conceptual Self-defense
Martial Arts After 40
Warrior Speed
The Martial Arts Training Diary for Kids
Teaching Martial Arts
Combat Strategy
The Art of Harmony
Total MindBody Training
1,001 Ways to Motivate Yourself and Others
Ultimate Fitness through Martial Arts
Taekwondo Kyorugi: Olympic Style Sparring

For more information:
Turtle Press
1-800-77-TURTL
e-mail: orders@turtlepress.com

http://www.turtlepress.com